THE PERMANENT WEIGHT LOSS PLAN

A 10 STEP APPROACH TO ENDING YO-YO DIETING

JANICE ASHER, MD,
AND
JAE RIVERA

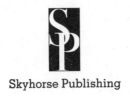

Skyhorse Publishing

Skyhorse Publishing books may be purchased in bulk at special discounts for sales promotion, corporate gifts, fund-raising, or educational purposes. Special editions can also be created to specifications. For details, contact the Special Sales Department, Skyhorse Publishing, 307 West 36th Street, 11th Floor, New York, NY 10018 or info@skyhorsepublishing.com.

Skyhorse® and Skyhorse Publishing® are registered trademarks of Skyhorse Publishing, Inc.®, a Delaware corporation.

Visit our website at www.skyhorsepublishing.com.

10 9 8 7 6 5 4 3 2 1

Library of Congress Cataloging-in-Publication Data

Names: Asher, Janice, author. | Rivera, Jae, author.
Title: The permanent weight loss plan: a 10 step approach to ending yo-yo dieting / Janice Asher, MD, and Jae Rivera.
Description: New York, NY: Skyhorse Publishing, [2020] | Includes bibliographical references and index.
Identifiers: LCCN 2019038932 (print) | LCCN 2019038933 (ebook) | ISBN 9781510751484 (trade paperback) | ISBN 9781510751491 (ebook)
Subjects: LCSH: Weight loss.
Classification: LCC RM222.2 .A832 2020 (print) | LCC RM222.2 (ebook) | DDC 613.2/5—dc23
LC record available at https://lccn.loc.gov/2019038932
LC ebook record available at https://lccn.loc.gov/2019038933

Cover design by Laura Klynstra

Printed in the United States of America

I dedicate this book to my patients who courageously shared their stories with me and who allowed me to help them create new ones.
—Janice

For everyone who needs proof that they are not an exception—it's absolutely possible for you, too.
—Jae

Contents

Preface

We are an older gynecologist and a younger badass anthropology PhD student who each lost a lot of weight in a healthy way and never gained it back. That's an achievement, and we'll show you what we learned in order to make that a reality.

But there's something even more important that we discovered and want to share with you in this book. We each learned, in our own ways, that self-loathing is a dead end and that kindness toward oneself is the starting point, not just the endpoint, of changing your relationship with food.

Please believe in yourself. Believe that you can do this, and believe that you deserve to do this.

You are not a happy, thin person stuck inside a sad, fat person. You are a person of value already. You will enhance your happiness by taking care of yourself physically and mentally. And when you do that, the weight loss will follow. We can help.

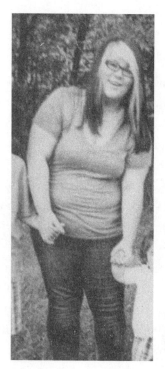

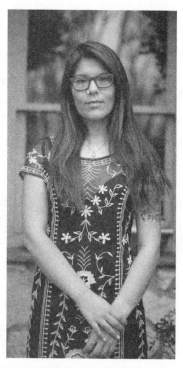

Jae, before   Jae, after © Tim Lee

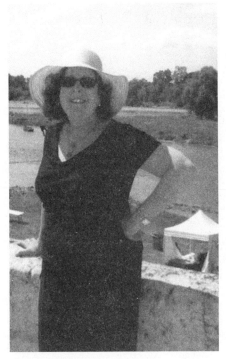

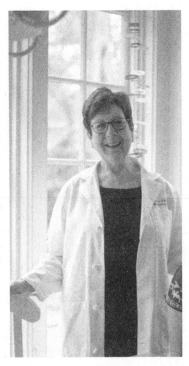

Janice, before

Janice, after © Tim Lee

INTRODUCTION

Hitting Bottom

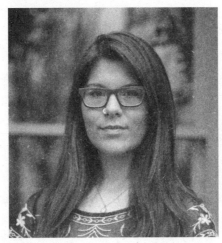

© Tim Lee

I am Jae.

It is the summer after my high school graduation, and I'm working at the local Pizza Hut. I'm physically exhausted, even though I've done very little physically. It's time to go, and I start to head out the door, but the manager stops me. Someone named Karen had ordered six pizzas, two orders of breadsticks, and a dessert stick, but she never bothered to show up, and they're mine if I want them. I've never met Karen, but at this moment, she is my new favorite person. I can't wait to drive home, descend to the basement, turn on Netflix, and eat myself happy.

I get home and check the freezer in the mudroom before entering the house. There's a half-gallon of ice cream, and better yet it's mint chocolate chip. I've just hit the trifecta—carbs, melted cheese, and ice cream. I stop only to tell my mom that I am home, avoiding the concern in her eyes. I imagine that she's holding herself back from saying anything. I know she wants what's best for me, but I wonder if maybe she thinks I'm just a lost cause. I go down the stairs and turn on the next episode of America's Next Top Model. The irony is completely lost on me as I open the containers and start eating mindlessly. In the next two hours, I consume ten breadsticks, four slices of pizza, and half of a half-gallon of ice cream. I see nothing wrong with this.

When I started college, I weighed 270 pounds. In my sophomore and junior years of college, I lost 142 pounds—52 percent of my body weight—through uncomplicated diet and exercise. I have successfully kept the weight off for over four years by evaluating and reevaluating my relationship with food and my body every day. If freshman Jae could see college graduate Jae today, she wouldn't believe her eyes.

I want to preface the rest of my experience by telling you that I am a scientist and an academic. It is my dream to become an expert in the field of human skeletal analysis. I want to be defined by my research and my friendships and relationships. I recognize that it's important for me to share my story so that you will know you are not alone and that you are capable of what you may think is impossible. Writing this book has been challenging for me, in that I learned it's hard for me to talk about my weight loss; not because I'm ashamed or embarrassed of myself or my body, but because it is not the focus of my life or a defining characteristic of my identity. I hope my experiences inspire you to make the choice to take care of your body and to love yourself.

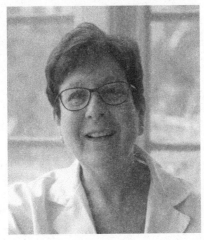

© Tim Lee

I am Janice.

I am on a stepladder, trying to reach into the back of the cabinet over the refrigerator. I am foraging for some old Halloween candy or anything else that's chocolate. I know that it will be uncomfortable coming down off the ladder because my knees hurt. I know that my knees hurt in part because I have gained weight—a lot of weight—and now weigh exactly what I had weighed when I was nine months pregnant. Just baby fat, right? Except that the baby is now twenty-three years old.

A single thought floats into my mind: You are pathetic. *And then, thank goodness, another thought replaces it:* This stops now. *And it did. That's the story I want to share with you.*

I am a gynecologist who lost 30 pounds. Thirty pounds—big deal, you say. Well, it is a big deal. It's a big deal because I'm in my sixties and had flunked every diet I'd ever been on. It's a big deal because I've kept the weight off for more than five years, which is something only a small fraction of people who lose weight can say.

It's a big deal because even though poor nutrition is the major cause of so many preventable diseases, I never learned much at all about healthy eating in medical school. So I had to develop my own strategies by reading all the

3

recent medical research and by personal trial and error. The strategies I used—and continue to use—have been helpful to many of my patients, and that's incredibly gratifying to me. Most of all, it's a big deal because I'm really proud of myself and happy to be living a life with less pain and more joy.

This is not a typical diet book. This book will not help you fit into those skinny pants in ten days. This is not a book about losing a certain amount of weight. Let us be clear: our ultimate goal is not about weight loss per se. Our ultimate goal is to help you to stop feeling shame about your body and to live a healthier life. We will provide you with tools for eating in a physically and emotionally healthy way, and we promise that the ultimate result will be sustainable weight loss.

The essence of this book is to help you redefine what it means to take care of yourself. Hating yourself is over. Hating your body is over. Saying mean things to yourself is over. The war between you and food is over.

This book is about eating without shame.

CHAPTER 1

Jae & Janice—We've Walked the Walk

> I thought to myself that I needed to lose just one pound, and then I could move on to the next one. If I started that day and lost one pound per week, then in a hundred weeks, I could be a hundred pounds lighter.

Jae's Story

In July of 2012, I went to see my physician for a routine physical before starting college the following month. The nurse led me down the hallway and asked me to remove my shoes and step on the scale. After a few moments, she announced "270," and I'm sure I didn't even bat an eye. Then, I went to the exam room, where the doctor told me she was concerned that I was class II morbidly obese and prediabetic. I was eighteen years old, and I wore size twenty pants, and I couldn't walk for more than a mile without my legs and feet hurting.

A month later, I packed my bags and said goodbye to my home for my new life at the University of Pennsylvania in Philadelphia. I had absolutely no idea what to expect about my time on the east coast—my hometown was small, rural, and anything but exciting. Now, I was about to land in the middle of one of the biggest cities in America. I was excited, but scared out of my mind.

Since my parents are teachers, they had to take me to Philadelphia well before the official move-in date so they could return home in time to start their own school year. This meant I had five days ahead of me when I could have explored the campus and the city, when I could have made friends with the other students who had also moved in before school started. Instead, I shut myself in my room, binge-watched nine seasons of Grey's Anatomy, *and finished off a week's worth of food in three days.*

Once new student orientation started, I had to leave my room. I went to a few school events, and it was immediately apparent to me that I did not look like anyone else at Penn. I felt embarrassed by the way people looked at me. I isolated myself. I tried not to eat in public or take extra food like everyone else did. I didn't want to be "that fat girl." Instead, I ate in secret or at night, once everyone else had gone out to parties.

You're supposed to have fun at college—go out, meet new people, make lifelong friends. I so much wanted to be the person who fearlessly introduces herself to everyone who crosses her path, but the reality was that I was not outgoing, and I was not confident. I was sure that no one looked past my looks.

Once classes started, I fell into a pretty solid routine, especially when it came to food. Before my 9:00 a.m. Spanish class, I ate two bagels loaded with cream cheese. Lunch was a chicken sandwich with cheese and bacon and a side of fries. Dinner in the dining hall was several pieces of pizza; no vegetables and no fruit. My real downfall was the unlimited access to the dessert tables and ice cream bar. I doubt there was a meal at the dining hall, including breakfast, that didn't end with ice cream.

I really could not have cared less about the "Freshman Fifteen"—those extra pounds that so many college students gain during their first year. I started college with ten times that much extra weight on my body, so what further damage could fifteen pounds do? In my mind, I had already lost the battle. My many past attempts at dieting and losing weight had failed. I was defeated, and I had accepted that I was never going to change. How could I even begin to motivate myself when I already constantly told myself that I was going to fail, just as I had done for what felt like two million times before?

Two moments during my first semester at Penn challenged this feeling of pessimism. When I started school, I ordered bright teal jeans in a size twenty, the color choice a part of my strategy to distract attention away from my body by redirecting it to the clothing itself. When I put these jeans on for the first time, they would not zip. I had gone past a size twenty, and I felt horrible.

The second and most powerful turning point for me was during an anthropology class. The professor showed a slide of two women's body scans (these scans take a picture of a "slice" of the person so doctors can visualize the internal structures). One woman was five-foot-six and weighed 120 pounds. The other woman was the same height, but she weighed 250 pounds. I remember how striking it was to see the body composition right there in front of me. I couldn't ignore it. I heard my classmates' shocked reactions to the picture, and all I could think about was the fact that I weighed twenty pounds more than the woman on the left. I couldn't believe I was doing this to my body.

I decided I was finally ready to change. Starting now.

I began by doing research on the online forum Reddit to learn more about weight loss. Through this, I found reddit.com/r/progresspics, where people post pictures of their transformations and tell their stories about how they approached weight loss. There were so many people who looked like me—people my age or my weight—who were losing twenty, forty, or a hundred-plus pounds! They shared the same thoughts and concerns about their bodies, weight loss, societal pressures, and other struggles (like binge eating) that I experienced. Provided with all these examples of people who were successful, I felt part of a community that understood my mental and physical struggles. I found a glimmer of hope.

That one glimmer was all I needed.

Now I knew that I wanted to look different, feel different, and move differently—but I had zero idea of how to get there. One night, I sat down at my desk and opened my yearly planner. I thought to myself that I needed to lose just one pound, and then I could move on to the next one. If I started that day and lost one pound per week, then in a hundred weeks, I could be a hundred pounds lighter. Of course, by then, I would be in my junior year of college. But I was going to be a junior in college no matter what, so did I want to stay the way I was, or did I want to change so I could have at least a year and a half left of a normal college experience, not to mention the rest of my life?

I chose the latter option. I wrote a large "1" in the top-right corner on the page for the week ahead. Then I wrote a "2" on the next page for the following week, and for each successive week, I increased the number by one until I hit a total of a hundred weeks. This was my benchmark for how I was going to keep myself focused on my ultimate goal.

What was important for me about this strategy was that it was a long-term approach, and it was not dramatic. I was not trying to crash diet. I was not trying to starve myself. But I also wanted my college years to be a time when I could feel pretty and confident, and go to parties if I wanted to. For me, this approach was the most realistic way to achieve my goals.

How was this different from the other times that I'd tried to lose weight? What changed was that my motivation and decision to lose weight had come from my own thought process. It was my own decision, instead of being a result of external pressure. I was motivated by wanting to fit into those teal pants and by the photo of the body scans from my anthropology class—and by a deeply rooted need to rid myself of the angry and hurtful thoughts that I carried with me at every moment.

I went back to Reddit for advice, tools, and suggestions to prepare myself to follow through on the commitment I had made. When I first started making changes in how I ate, I knew absolutely nothing about nutrition and fitness. Many people on /r/progresspics used an app called MyFitnessPal to track and count their calorie intake. I downloaded it to begin to understand how many calories I was actually consuming. This was one of the most important points in my journey—I am a very visual person, and MyFitnessPal showed me why I was gaining weight so rapidly (about twenty pounds per year throughout high school). It was clear that I could not lose weight by eating over three thousand calories a day. That first semester, I made small changes, taking apples from the dining hall instead of ice cream or making a turkey sandwich instead of eating a huge burger and fries. It was a slow start, but I was determined to change my eating patterns in a way that was right for me.

During the summer after my freshman year in 2013, I lived in an apartment with four other students, one of whom was an avid bicyclist and enthusiastic Philadelphia explorer. I got my own bike and began to see the city with him. This made it hard to make my nightly trips to the local convenience store. Instead of eating whenever I wanted for emotional reasons, I began to learn how to eat in intervals and in realistic portion sizes. I constantly reminded myself that it had taken years to put on all this weight, and that it was going to take some time to get it back off.

Everyone in my apartment that summer was a vegetarian, and I decided to give it a try. Honestly, meat was expensive and I didn't mind an excuse to save money. Up until then, I was a big fan of fast and convenient food, and the only vegetables I would touch were peas, carrots, corn, and cauliflower (and even then, only if they were drowned in melted cheese). Being vegetarian meant that eating from fast-food restaurants just did not work anymore. During that time, healthy fast-casual restaurants and healthy options on fast-food menus were not yet widely available. I was forced to try new foods, and I learned to love all vegetables. I remember so vividly the first time I tried Brussels sprouts at lunch in the Penn Museum cafe. They were roasted with garlic and rosemary and were unforgettable. My housemates and I celebrated my first meat-free week with vegetarian falafel, and I loved it!

I soon ordered my first pair of jean shorts from Old Navy and wore them in public. They were a size sixteen, and I was so proud. I went from an XL shirt down to a large. I finally had tangible proof that I was taking steps in a positive direction. This was for real; I was actually doing this. That first summer, I lost only 20 of the 142 pounds that I would eventually lose, but I wanted to keep the good changes going. MyFitnessPal became my primary tool for weight loss. I was committed to conscientiously logging calories and had learned about portion sizes in the process. I learned to calculate how many calories I needed daily to maintain weight, and thus how many calories I could eat daily to lose weight each week. I was confident I could stick with this because I was approaching weight loss in a healthy way.

At some point in the fall of my sophomore year, my roommate asked me to join her at the gym and I thought, "Why not? What do I have to lose?" I barely lasted twenty minutes on the elliptical machine. It felt like hell, and I didn't go back, but I remember feeling so proud of myself for trying. In January 2014, I was ready to start something new. Many people in /r/progresspics often talked about how running had changed their lives. Specifically, I noticed that they mentioned a program called "C25K" or "Couch to 5K." The eight-week program uses interval training to help a person who typically cannot run for more than a minute at a time to eventually run an entire five-kilometer (3.1 mile) stretch. I decided to go for it.

My friend Sarah decided to try it, too, and I honestly couldn't have done it without her. She kept me accountable, which made a huge impact on my ability to succeed. We went to the gym together and ran at the same time. I knew I would feel guilty if I wasn't doing my part, so I had *more motivation to show up to our runs. If we weren't able to go to the gym together, we had to send a picture of our feet on the treadmill to each other as proof that we were still doing the workout! Despite having an accountability partner, it was still hard for me. Going to the gym as a fat person is incredibly intimidating, something I talk about in more detail in Chapter 19.*

Completing the C25K program was one of the hardest things I've ever done. It was not only physically, but also mentally, challenging. I had to keep running even when I could see the fat jiggle up and down in my stomach and legs. It was embarrassing enough to run by myself, and now other people could see me, too? Damn, it was so emotionally tough! The important thing, though, is that even though there were times when I felt like crap, I did it. And was I aware with each training run that I was truly instituting an entire lifestyle change? Hell, no! I was taking it just one run or one workout at a time.

By July 2014, I had lost a hundred pounds. I left to study abroad in Australia, and I made another pivotal decision on the plane. I realized that I was susceptible to the common "study abroad" experience of gaining ten pounds or so, and that if I did, I would have to restart my weight loss plan all over again when I returned home. Or, I could just stay aware and focused enough while abroad to maintain my weight. At that moment, I also saw a third option: I could take the next six months to keep on my weight loss path and come back to America a lighter, fitter person. I chose the third option.

I lost another twenty-five pounds in Australia. I continued my healthy habits when I returned to the University of Pennsylvania and completed the rest of my junior year. In the summer of 2015, I stepped on the scale and read the numbers. I had lost 142 pounds—52 percent of what I had weighed when I had started at Penn three years before!

I had done it. In the span of just two years, I had transformed my life.

Jae—in Janice's Words

Like all my patients, Jae was a student at the University of Pennsylvania, where I was the director of Women's Health at the Student Health Service. She sat across from me, so quiet and soft-spoken but clearly incredibly intelligent. I did a double take when I looked at her chart and saw that she'd lost more than fifty pounds in the last year. Then I learned that she'd lost almost a hundred pounds before that.

"How did you lose all that weight?" I asked.

"Diet and exercise," she replied.

That's all she said, as though it were a simple answer to a simple question. I pressed for more details, telling her that I was personally and professionally interested in the subject. "I decided that I needed to change, and I found a way to do it, so I did," Jae told me. "And if I can do it, I think I can help other people do it, too." She added that she was thinking about writing a book about her experience.

"I'm also thinking about writing a book about healthy weight loss," I told her. "After you graduate, would you like to write one together?" And so began our collaboration.

Since then, I've come to be even more impressed by Jae's intelligence and modesty. When Jae invited me to attend her graduation ceremony in the Department of Anthropology, I found out for the first times at the ceremony that Jae had 1) graduated magna cum laude and Phi Beta Kappa, and 2) won the prize for the best senior thesis. Even then, she didn't mention that her thesis was more than 150 pages long!

Jae will never tell you how special she is—so that honor falls to me. I am thrilled to be sharing authorship of this book with such an amazing young woman.

Janice's Story

My story is much shorter and less dramatic than Jae's. I didn't really have a weight problem until I was forty, after the birth of my second baby.

Even as I write that, I remember that I'd always thought I was a little overweight, or at least flabby—certainly "imperfect," as I thought at the time—even when I was a size six or eight. I had always had a sweet tooth and ate large portions, though I managed to get away with it when I was younger. My mother was a fabulous baker, and Friday was her baking day. When I'd come home from school every Friday, there would be two pies sitting on the counter: one for the family and one just for me. My pie was smaller—but not that small! I'd eat the whole thing right there and then.

I never enjoyed exercise, either. When I was a teenager, girls didn't have to participate in gym if we had our period. My gym teachers never seemed to notice (or maybe pretended not to notice, since I was so pathetic at sports) that I seemed to have my period just about every week.

Somehow, I got away with these habits. Until I didn't. My second baby was a year old and I still couldn't fit into anything except my maternity clothes. My age and my changing metabolism had caught up with me, and I had no idea what to do. Don't get me wrong—I knew full well what I "should" eat. I would try one diet or another, and it would work for a while. Until it didn't.

I've been a gynecologist for forty years, and in that time, I've taken care of thousands of women. I would estimate that I have met fewer than a dozen who were happy with their bodies. That's crazy—but it's also true. And it was true of me, too. I hated my body, and I felt like a total hypocrite: I would spend all day counseling patients about the importance of healthy eating and regular exercise—and most of all, about the importance of stopping this body-shaming nonsense. Then, I would go home and eat chocolate and cookies and end up feeling disgusted with how I felt and embarrassed by how I looked. Whatever words I was saying about food and exercise weren't helping me, and they weren't helping my patients, either. What good does it do to tell someone that "calories-in/calories-out" is a simple equation? What good does it do to tell someone that they should exercise? How do those words help someone with motivation, optimism, strategies, and changes in behavior that can be sustained? The answer is, they don't.

Then I had that moment on the stepladder, and something within me clicked: it was the realization that being angry with myself was not going to motivate me to change in a sustainable way, but that wanting to take good care of my body would help with the weight. I decided to shift my thinking. I would think about being more active with my daughters and with my future grandchildren. I would think about being able to live an independent and vigorous life as an old lady. I was going to make more space in my brain by not playing the endless loop in my head about what I wanted to eat but shouldn't eat—or shouldn't have eaten that now made me feel ashamed and undisciplined and hopeless.

Once I reframed "wanting to lose weight" into a new paradigm of "wanting to take care of myself," the day-to-day strategies fell into place. I gave myself constant, gushy, positive feedback. I got rid of all the chocolate I had in the house. I weighed myself every day. I started every meal with vegetables. I planned ahead for what I was going to eat at the next snack and at the next meal. I share these strategies in greater detail in the pages ahead.

I also tried out my ideas with patients who were struggling with being overweight and who were open to trying something new. Together, we would devise short-term and long-term goals that were achievable and sustainable. These were emotional goals as much as they were behavioral. It had to be a positive experience! I was moved and excited by how many of these young women were able to make significant changes, not just in their weight, but more importantly in how they thought about themselves and their bodies.

Along with a nutritionist and a therapist at the Student Health Service, I started an education/support group for students who were struggling with issues related to being heavy. We never talked about actual weights or calorie counts. Instead, we talked about changing our relationship with food. Every week for six weeks, these students shared their frustrations, their struggles, and their shame. But by the end of those six weeks, their mindsets had shifted dramatically. They began to learn that feeling good about themselves would result in, not result from, weight loss. They began to learn and create their own strategies, which I also share in the course of this book.

Then, Jae came to see me; and the rest, as they say, is history. Since that time, our relationship has vastly deepened. Jae and I are now close friends and cowriters. She has launched herself into a career as an anthropologist, and we relate to each other as trusted and valued colleagues. She has enriched my life immeasurably.

Janice—in Jae's Words

Have you ever just walked into a room and felt safe? That there's a shield around you and that nothing bad can touch you? It's as if the walls you've spent your whole life constructing suddenly have no purpose, and you can put aside your baseline anxiety for the moment.

I've rarely felt that kind of safety, but I did the moment Janice walked into the exam room. It was like the air had changed. She asked me many questions, but I never felt judged. She treated me like someone she had cared about her whole life, even though she had just met me.

Janice asked me about my weight loss, which I had brought up only because I thought it might be related to the reason I was sitting in front of her that day. "It was just diet and exercise," I answered, because that's really just what it was. I saw my weight loss as something that had happened because it needed to happen, but Janice saw something different.

Her reaction inspired me to reconsider my view of what I had accomplished. She mentioned she wanted to write a book about weight loss and asked if I was interested in writing it with her after I graduated. I was in disbelief that she would even be interested in my story. I didn't think the obstacles I'd overcome were special compared to what so many people out there had achieved.

From then on, every time I spoke to Janice about my weight loss or the things I faced in my life, she responded with encouragement and love. This was new to me. For so long, I had felt like I was in an uphill battle. People praised me for my academic achievements, but those nagging voices in the back of my head always urged me to brush them off. But Janice didn't let me off the hook. She drilled it into me, over and over: I had accomplished something worth celebrating; I had earned the praise. She made me feel that I deserved to feel proud of myself.

Janice is made of love that is stitched together with kindness. When you stand next to her, it's impossible not to see and feel her love for others, for her kids, and for just about anyone who brings positivity and kindness into the world.

STEP ONE:

Appreciate Your Body before You Lose Even a Single Ounce

CHAPTER 2

Your Goals Are within Reach—But Not in the Way You've Been Told

> The key to sustainable weight loss is not "willpower" and deprivation—it's kindness toward yourself and letting go of shame.

The Shame Stops Today

Diet books, weight loss promoters, and other "experts" will tell you that self-discipline and even deprivation are the keys to weight loss success. They claim that once you lose weight, you'll live happily ever after and never, ever regain the weight or feel ashamed of your body. Of course, that's not true. What actually happens is that most people tend to reach their maximum weight loss after six months or so[1] and then gradually regain the weight (and often end up weighing more than they did in the first place) over a period of one to five years.[2]

Why does this happen? There are many explanations, based largely on the body's adaptation to weight loss—and *not* on all the reasons people give for blaming others and blaming themselves for regaining the weight.

The two of us are among only 20 percent of people who have successfully achieved long-term weight loss,[3] and we want to help you join our club. We'll share with you our strategies that are backed up by actual science rather than marketing ploys, and we'll also share our personal secrets to success.

We disagree with the so-called experts. The key to sustainable weight loss is not "willpower" and deprivation—it's kindness toward yourself and letting go of shame. You want to lose weight and keep it off? You want to change your emotional relationship with food? If that's what you want, **the shame stops today. No, not when you lose weight. Today.**

We suggest that your mother, your doctor, and the sponsors of those ads showing smiling skinny people holding up the waistbands of their fat jeans have it exactly backward. We suggest you need to *start* with letting go of the shame about your eating and your body. If you do that, then you will be able to carry out a strategy that will *result* in weight loss that can be sustained for the rest of your life.

Let's start with this premise: **you are already worth taking care of.** Your scale measures only your weight, not your worth. In our culture, heavy people are viewed as undisciplined or unmotivated. Please don't be part of that appallingly cruel and wrong-headed kind of thinking. Fat-shaming other people is wrong; and fat-shaming yourself is wrong, too. Emotional eating and shame are tightly interconnected, and that connection can be broken. Let us be clear: breaking this connection does not happen by beating yourself up. Beating yourself up leads to one failed diet after another, as well as to the feeling that *you're* the one who failed, not the poorly designed diet. Overcoming shame, on the other hand, happens when you change the way you think about yourself and talk to yourself. We propose to you a sustainable, permanent lifestyle change that results from kindness and knowledge. Let us explain.

How Eating Becomes Emotional

Before you can really grapple with emotional eating and your relationship with food, it's good to understand where it begins. It starts early: food is love. Almost all of us have experience with that notion. You had a bad day at school? Your mom baked your favorite gooey brownies. What made holidays so special? The food, of course! Yes, you're looking forward to getting together with your family, but what you may be thinking about the most is getting together with your grandmother's pumpkin pie, the Christmas tamales and hot chocolate, the Chanukah potato pancakes. We could go on and on. From the beginning, we are taught that food is fun and happiness and stress relief and family and connection.

That was the start of emotional eating. But something more sinister followed in its path. Kids called you fat. Parents, probably unknowingly, said something insensitive or even cruel. Maybe you were told it was "just teasing." Maybe it was a hurtful, critical comment that was made "for your own good."

This is when you began to learn about shame.

This shame was only reinforced as you got older, as our fat-shaming society pressured you to be conscious and critical of your body and to measure your attractiveness by some arbitrary standard of beauty, where stick-thin models look like they're starving. Now, as an adult, you no longer need anyone else to make you feel shame. You have learned all the lessons and can do it all by yourself. The damage has been done—no one can make you feel more awful about yourself than you can. It's only natural that your response to the internalized shame is to want to comfort yourself. And what has your go-to comfort always been? We don't need to tell you—here you are, reading this book.

We need to emphasize this point: **You are not to blame for using emotional eating as a coping mechanism.** There is no way that, as a child, you could have foreseen that eating in this way would have so many physical and emotional consequences. Now that you're an adult, you still carry your childhood wounds and comfort-seeking responses within you. Unfortunately, emotional eating is an attempt to fill a hole that cannot be filled. You literally "swallow your pain." But here's the good news: you do not need to be defined by these wounds.

The Antidote to Shame is Kindness

If you want to move away from the shame that you're feeling, you need to make a commitment to kindness. This commitment makes the process not only positive, but also permanent. If you're willing to commit to kindness and compassion toward yourself, then we can show you how to commit to changing the way you eat and the way you think about food.

Yes, we know this may sound like a simplistic idea; but we swear, it is not. Being kind to yourself instead of berating yourself will help you get started and will also be the end result of the process. It does not mean that you attempt to turn your body into one that looks like a fashion model's (which is likely to be dangerously thin, anyway). It doesn't mean that you're never going to backslide and eat a bunch of junk food when you're feeling low. There will be times when it may seem like you are losing your way. A commitment to treating yourself with kindness simply means that even if you do veer from your path, that detour will be only temporary if you continue to live your life in a way in which you are compassionate toward yourself.

Let's put it this way: losing weight will not make you love yourself, but loving yourself will certainly help you lose weight. That may sound sappy or even selfish, but it's not—it's just true.

Jae's Path from Emotional Eating

Jae—I want to share my own personal experience with the effects of out-of-control eating. I hope to show you that your interaction with food does not make you weird or defective. It is what it is, and there are strategies to help you overcome your obstacles.

My mother was raised in a household where delicious food treats were emotional and financial indulgences. When she had her own kids, my mother was determined to do things differently. If I asked for a treat, like the chocolate-covered Rice Krispies bar from the local coffee shop, she would say yes because it represented emotional and financial freedom for her. "Indulgent" foods became routine parts of my diet, and they were associated with happy feelings and comfort. When things were tough for me, food became my emotional crutch. So, is it any surprise that once I started getting bullied in middle school and once the stress of high school studies kicked in, I turned to food as my coping mechanism?

When I think back to my time in high school. I honestly can't remember any time I experienced hunger. I was eating at 7 a.m., 10 a.m., 11:30 a.m., 2:30 p.m., 5 p.m., and 8 p.m.—there was no time for my body to even digest what I had eaten a few hours before. I was on a constant cycle of putting food in my mouth, and it didn't matter what it was. I would have had breakfast and a snack and lunch and a Subway Footlong after school, and I would still eat two servings of pasta and chips and dessert once I got home. My issue was that food was not for sustenance; it was for comfort, a way to fill a void that was utterly irrational.

In college, when my nutritionist told me to just have one cookie at my college dorm's cookie night, I felt so unheard and invalidated. How did she not understand that there was no way for me to just have just one when there were four hundred more waiting to be eaten? If my nutritionist didn't understand my disordered relationship with food, neither did my therapist, who said, "If you're going to have a cookie, have the best cookie you can find, in your favorite flavor, and make sure it counts so you can savor it." The problem was she was still working under the assumption that I could limit myself to just one cookie. My nutritionist and therapist both focused on the concept of practicing self-restraint, as though I could be rational in those situations, but that's not how my brain works. When I eat, my brain turns off and rational thinking is out the door. I am in pure primal brain—food to mouth, chew, swallow, repeat.

*It took me a long time to accept that I am not a failure just because my brain and body don't act in the same way as other people's. **I'm not broken; I just work differently.***

A commitment to kindness is not the same as that ludicrously overused term, *self-esteem*. We're not telling you to whisper sweet nothings in your own ear about what a goddess or god you are. We're not pretending that discipline, perseverance, or even struggle are not part of the process. It's going to be hard to forego the ice cream you want, to order salad instead of fries, or to put on your sneakers and go for a walk. This is hard! If it were as simple as "eat less, move more," then two-thirds of the population in the United States would not be overweight or obese! Here's our solemn promise to you: it won't be as hard as listening to the self-critical voice in your head that harangues you all day long—sometimes softly in the background, sometimes front and center—but always there and always cruel.

What's the problem with negative thoughts? Aren't they useful? Sometimes, yes. Humankind has been able to survive as well as it has partly because people are hardwired to pay attention to negative experiences so they can quickly escape danger. This is perhaps one reason why negative thoughts and experiences tend to have a lasting impact on us in a way that positive ones seldom do. It takes far greater awareness and effort to focus on what is positive and then to sustain that focus.

Can't negative thoughts motivate us to do better? Well, yes, they may have their function in the short term. You may need your inner boot camp sergeant to get you out of bed on a cold, rainy morning. Ultimately, though, negative thoughts are self-defeating. They end up making you feel even worse about yourself. And, as we've seen, how do you respond to feeling bad? By turning to your source of solace: food.

Don't Believe Everything You Think

Here's another thing about negative thoughts: usually, they're not even true! The term "fake it 'til you make it" may be a huge asset for you in this journey. Instead of allowing your head to be filled with awful thoughts about all the things that are wrong or bad about yourself, you can learn to replace them with thoughts and statements that are positive. The more you practice this, the easier it becomes. The best part is when you realize that the positive statements are actually more credible than the negative ones, and that you're not faking it at all.

Janice—*For me, the most important and meaningful change has not been ridding myself of excess weight, but rather ridding myself of the self-loathing tape that was on a continuous loop inside my head. There is only one response to shame that makes any sense to me: kindness and compassion toward oneself. It is this change, and not just the weight loss, that has made me feel great—and that is why I have not gained back weight. I simply don't want to go back to being so self-critical.*

Let us explain what we mean by using pretending, or "faking it," to change your thoughts from self-critical to kind. Imagine that you are with your best friend. We're assuming you're a good person, and you know how to be a good friend. When your best friend is feeling like crap because someone had given her "constructive criticism" that her dress was looking a bit tight, you're not going to say, "Oh yes, I see what they mean—you've kind of let yourself go a bit." Hell, no! If your other friend was "on a diet" or "on a cut" and ate three donuts, you wouldn't try to make him feel even worse about it. Instead, you might say that he had a crazy, stressful moment and sought relief in a totally understandable way. It doesn't mean that he's a failure, or weak, or pathetic. Instead, you're more likely to tell him that life can be tough and that donuts can taste awfully good.

When your friends are feeling sad and hurt, you intuitively know to speak kindly to emphasize their strengths and point out the things that make them valuable and that make the friendship valuable to you. So, why would you speak to yourself any differently? Why would you call yourself a failure or weak or pathetic? It's time to drop the double standard. You have to live with yourself forever, so why not make sure you like—and respect—the company? When you say hurtful things to yourself, stop and think about it. Would you ever look someone in the eye and say those terrible things?

How about talking to yourself as you would talk to your good friend? When you get stuck, think of what you would say to your best friend—in essence, *change the script.* Scolding yourself and belittling yourself do not work. Hating yourself cannot be an option if you want to move forward. Expressions of self-negativity not only hurt you on an individual level, but they also hurt the other people in your life who you care about. Negativity is contagious; it makes others feel bad, sad, and more negative. Being around all that negativity just reinforces the cycle of feeling bad about yourself. Positivity, on the other hand, is also contagious, a gift that you will both give and receive. By opening your heart to yourself, it will become so much easier to open your heart to the world, with the result being an increase in compassion and optimism toward others. And that compassion will return to you as well.

Jae—It became so clear to me that I couldn't perpetuate change with negativity. Negativity is what got me to a bad point; it's what fueled the voices in my head and distorted my true sense of worth; it's what surrounded me when I was among groups of people, or looking at myself in the mirror, or moving my hand for that third cupcake. I don't make room for that negativity anymore. Positivity means I've made a conscious choice to accept myself in all forms, to make myself healthier, and to love who I am. I have post-it notes surrounding my mirror that are filled with positive affirmations and the aspects of myself that I'm proud of. The script has changed.

Ultimately, you have total control over only one thing: your thoughts. Some of these thoughts about yourself are unnecessarily cruel, and many of them are probably untrue. Challenge these negative thoughts! Then, replace them with kinder, more positive, and, most likely, more *accurate* thoughts!

You Deserve This

Please be clear that this is the decision you are making because you *want* to make it. Honestly, wanting it isn't even enough on its own—you also need to acknowledge that this is a commitment to prioritizing your own needs. Does that sound selfish? It's not. We are all responsible for caring for ourselves. If you're healthier, more energetic, and happier, then you're going to be way better at caring for others. The wonderful psychologist and meditation teacher Tara Brach writes, "This revolutionary act of treating ourselves tenderly can begin to undo the aversive messages of a lifetime."[4]

You can choose to live in a space where you aren't at war with food and your body. You deserve this, and so do the people in your life whom you love. You deserve to care enough about yourself to make this commitment. You cannot reach your best self with negativity, guilt, and shame. Your body deserves respect and compassion right now.

We would like to offer you this: starting now, food and shame will no longer live together. We will help you want to eat and move in a physically and emotionally healthy way. You will not say mean things to yourself. You will not call yourself a failure. You will not see yourself as weak. You will not think that you are lacking "willpower."

The big question of this book is simple: Aren't you tired of feeling bad about yourself?

CHAPTER 3

Transforming Your Wishes into Reality

Let's be real: how has beating
yourself up worked out for you so far?

Suppose you have a goal of losing fifty pounds. What does that goal actually mean? Unless you lay the groundwork, saying your goal is to lose fifty pounds is like a Miss America contestant saying her goal is for world peace. Neither "goal" reflects the strategies and behaviors that will help you achieve your objectives. Having said that, goals really *are* important. In fact, goal-setting is one of the key components in helping people achieve their desired outcomes. In this chapter, we will help you create your own personal strategies for achieving specific and meaningful goals.

From dream to reality—that's what it's all about, isn't it? You go from wishing for weight loss to achieving the goal of actually losing—and *sustaining*—that loss. Sounds easy enough—but you know it isn't that simple. If it was, then everyone would be slim and fit. But we *promise* that you can be slimmer, fitter, and more content with yourself and your relationship to food and your body. There is in fact a proven path to get positive results—the two of us have taken every step ourselves (along with a few detours!), and we'll show you the way. Here are the three stops on your journey:

Thoughts –> Action –> Results

A study of overweight women found that participants were more successful at achieving their goal of losing weight when they strengthened the path that led from "cognition" (**thoughts**) to "behavior" (**action**) and then to "outcome" (**results**).[1] This is different from the advice that many "experts" give overweight people, which is to focus only on the desired result: weight loss. The problem is that by focusing just on the end result, you leave out the really important stuff: the *specific steps* you need to take to achieve that goal and to *stay* there. We're going to show you how to use **thoughts** to create the strategy for **action**. The impact of your actions will then be attaining the **results** you desire. In the remainder of this chapter, we'll focus on laying the foundation for your success: your thoughts.

Your Thoughts: They're All in Your Head

The first step is *cognition*—thoughts or awareness. In this context, cognition means thinking (and even writing) about the importance of changing your relationship with food, your strengths, your challenges, and your supports. At each step of the way, we'll help you develop strategies to get you through a particular situation.

If you're reading this book, then we can all agree that you're unhappy about the way you eat and about the effect that unhealthy habits and patterns are having on your life. That's the starting point. The next step is to think about—and write down—the reasons you want to change your relationship with food. In fact, we are going to ask you to write out several lists.

Why? When an idea is in your head, it often stops there. How many times have you solved one of the World's Greatest Problems while washing your hair in the shower, only to forget that solution by the time you reach for the towel? Writing helps you transform thoughts, feelings, and ideas into something tangible. You can look back on the words you wrote and consider them, add to them, or reframe them. And then *act* on them.

List #1: The Reasons You Want to Lose Weight

In her book *The Complete Beck Diet for Life*,[2] cognitive therapist Judith Beck suggests making a list of all the reasons you want to lose weight. We agree this is a great idea, and we urge you to write your own list, for several reasons:

- First, positive motivation will be a powerful force in this process of changing your relationship with food. Thinking about your list of why you want to lose weight, then adding to it and referring to it often, will greatly reinforce that motivation.
- Second, in the not-too-distant future, an unwelcome voice in your head, which we will call your "**Evil Twin**," is likely say, "To hell with this healthy eating stuff." You need to have a ready response. Your list will help you.
- Third, your list will help you track your progress. You will discover patterns, such as stress eating, emotional eating (sadness, anger), and situational eating (car, movies, television). Recognizing these patterns will help you to overcome challenges as they occur and to develop new patterns that will work for you, both physically and emotionally.

Janice's list:

- *I want to feel confident when I walk into a room filled with strangers.*
- *I want to be able to hike with my daughters.*
- *I want to feel proud of being in charge of my choices.*
- *I want to fit into those gorgeous, overpriced pants I bought two years ago.*
- *I want my knees and hips to feel happier.*
- *I want to enjoy shopping for clothes—not just accessories!*
- *I want to be able to run for a bus.*
- *I want to feel okay about someone taking a picture of me.*
- *I want to end up being a fit old lady who doesn't need to go to a nursing home.*
- *I want to set a good example for my patients.*

I can't overstate how important it was for me to write this list and have it readily accessible. Whenever I was discouraged or felt "discipline fatigue," I referred back to it to get me back on the motivation track. In fact, I still do.

Jae's list:

- *I want to accept and admire all of myself.*
- *I want actual evidence that I have the strength and self-discipline to accomplish my goals.*
- *I want to be an inspiration to myself and other people.*
- *I want to walk more than a mile without my knees and feet hurting.*
- *I want to go an entire day without having to readjust my clothes.*
- *I want to look in the mirror and smile.*
- *I want to be an example for my younger siblings of what it means to be strong and independent.*

- *I want to grow old without diabetes, cardiovascular disease, or any other preventable chronic diseases.*
- *If my partner and I ever decided to have children in the future, I would want to ensure that I can have a healthy pregnancy and a healthy baby.*

I need this list most when I'm feeling defeated and down. Having a prepared list of ideas and goals that mean a lot to me is something that sets me up to respond in a way that works.

Notice that our lists of motivators are **specific**. Yes, "I want to be thinner" may be a reason for losing weight, but it's not concrete enough and will not be very helpful. Make a list that helps you envision—and then act upon—the potential of a different future that you can create for yourself. For example, "I want to be able to walk a mile with my friends" is both more precise and motivating than "I want to get more exercise."

Our lists are also **positive**. We have deliberately avoided writing things like, "I want to stop hating my body." We urge you to leave your self-critical, negative voice behind. Let's be real: how has beating yourself up worked out for you so far?

With that in mind, realize that the time to write your list is not at the end of a bad day, after your train home was an hour late or the washing machine broke down. The time to make this list is right now—when you're feeling calm and optimistic about your ability to make changes that will truly enhance your life. Once you've got all your reasons on paper, pause and think about each one of them. Envision yourself as more confident, more energetic, and more self-accepting. What will that feel like? This is a crucial step because this vision is what will keep you going when you're ready to give up or when you've had a setback. Holding the idea

33

of a more vibrant version of yourself will be an incredibly valuable source of inspiration.

Janice—Several of my patients have told me that what helped them most was to write letters to themselves. These letters enabled them to step aside from themselves, to be more objective and compassionate, and to observe changes in their thought processes over time.

Deactivate Your Evil Twin

We hope that making this list has helped you to feel excited about the future and ready to do what it takes. But let's be real. Soon, maybe even as soon as the very next time you're hungry, you're going to hear from that self-defeating, critical, nasty voice in your head—your Evil Twin.

"To hell with this health crap," it says.

Or, "Just one cookie."

Or, "I've had such a miserable day—I deserve a burger and fries."

Or, "I'll do this when the stress in my life is over."

Your Evil Twin is not your friend. It only knows how to tell you all of the reasons why you can't become a better version of yourself. Your Evil Twin is a threat to your success—but not if you don't give it permission! And how do you deny it permission? Have you ever been in an argument where someone says something offensive, and your mind goes blank, only to have the *perfect* comeback come to mind later that day? We want you to have those comebacks ready *now*, so that you'll be prepared the next time your Evil Twin tries to sabotage your efforts. What do you say to the self-defeating voice in your head?

List #2: Rebuttal List for Your Evil Twin

Janice's list:

- *No matter what I'm feeling, chocolate is not going to make it better.*
- *I may be having a bad day, but unhealthy eating will just make a bad day worse, and I'd rather do something that will truly make the day better.*
- *You, Evil Twin, are not a trustworthy voice. I believe what I wrote on my list of why I want to eat differently.*

Jae's list:

- *There are enough unkind people in the world. I do not need to be my own bully.*
- *To hell with this? No! To hell with being fat and hating myself.*
- *I'm not going to give space to the mean voices in my head anymore. I am making the choice to fill my mind with positive messages and positive reinforcement.*
- *I am more than this piece of food.*
- *I did not get fat overnight, and I will not get healthy overnight, either. This takes patience and commitment, and I will see the results in a few weeks.*
- *Food is fuel. It does not hold emotional power.*

Notice in our lists that we are responding to the Evil Twin with confidence and resolve, not self-loathing and defeat. That positive, optimistic attitude is a dramatic departure from how we have talked to ourselves in the past. It represents a **paradigm shift**, i.e., a fundamental rejection of the negative assumptions we have held and a move toward new ways of thinking.

List #3: Shift the Paradigm

Once you've listed your responses to the Evil Twin, how do you really convince yourself of their truth? That's where the paradigm shift comes into play. Paradigm shifts allow us to reframe old negative, disparaging thoughts into positive thoughts that are just as real.

Here's what's worked for us:

Old Paradigm	New Paradigm
I deserve a cookie.	I deserve to feel good about myself.
Food is my friend, and I can use a friend right now.	A real friend doesn't make me feel horrible about myself.
I don't have time to exercise.	I deserve to make time to take care of myself.
I hate my body.	I am alive and vertical, and I thank my body for that. I'm excited about taking better care of myself.
I'm stuck this way forever.	I have the knowledge and power to take charge and live the life I have chosen.
It's too expensive to join a gym.	I'm going to find creative ways to meet challenges.

Now it's your turn to list the ways you can shift your paradigms. What do you tell yourself that is keeping you from making positive changes? How can you reframe a challenge to make it workable for you?

Customize Your Goals

Be sure that you choose goals that will work for *you*—and are therefore more likely to be achievable—not some notion of what your goals *should* be. Someone else's goal to be a size zero or to have "six-pack abs" or to climb Mount Everest has nothing to do with goals that are meaningful to you. If a goal isn't realistic, given the constraints of your schedule, responsibilities, and other needs, then you're just setting yourself up for failure.

Jae—Don't try something blindly just because someone else said to do it. Is it something that is truly realistic for you? For example, when I was trying to eat healthier foods while I was putting myself through college, someone recommended that I order meals from a food delivery service and eat that food exclusively. However, many of those meal subscription plans cost sixty dollars for just ten meals—an amount that was more than my grocery budget for the entire week! Instead, I spent some time looking up good recipes and learning what kinds of healthy substitutions I could make, and I found ways to incorporate these into my existing meal prep plans.

Another example is I have friends who have offered to be my gym buddies, which was very thoughtful and supportive of them. However, what they left out was that their gym cost eighty dollars for only four visits! I don't have that kind of money to spend at the gym. Instead, I make a conscious effort to go outside and run, walk, or hike on trails, and sometimes I invite friends to join me. I don't want to set myself up for failure.

Janice—It took me quite a while to realize that my goal to be the same size and shape I was before I had children was absurd—at least for me. Part of my process was to evolve to a place of being satisfied with and grateful for a body that was as fit and functional as possible.

Finally, your goals are not written in stone. Don't be afraid to change them. You might find over time that some goals no longer work well for you or are no longer relevant. Maybe you no longer care about running a marathon or fitting into your old prom dress. It makes sense to review your goals periodically to ensure that you're keeping yourself on track in a way that works for you. That's why we encourage you to write them down so you can refer back to them.

How Does It Feel to Be Optimistic?

At this point, take some time to review what you've done so far. Just sit with yourself, look over your list, and think about (or even better, write down) how it feels to know you have made the decision to take care of yourself. Honestly, have you felt this optimistic in a long time? Don't forget this feeling. This will be the feeling that will "feed" you and keep you motivated.

STEP TWO:

Choose Abundance over Deprivation

CHAPTER 4

You Are What You Eat

The good news is there are concrete and specific actions you can take to lessen the influence of ever-present unhealthy processed foods . . . the two of us are living proof!

Maybe you've already tried too many diets to count—low-fat, low-carb, paleo, juice fast, whatever. It may be the same story each time: this time, the diet will work; this time your willpower will triumph. You might do wonderfully at first, but then what? You go through a stressful time, and you find yourself derailed; or the weight loss is slow, and you feel discouraged. Perhaps you just get tired of the whole thing.

A "well-meaning" person might ask, "Are you sure you want to eat that?" and you go crazy. *Forget it!* you think. Here you are, trying your best, and someone piles on the criticism anyway. So you give up the diet, which feels like you're giving up on yourself. You feel defeat, maybe shame. By now, you may have lost and gained a hundred pounds by repeating this cycle. You wonder, *What's the point?*

Janice—Here's my new favorite term that I learned from my college-age patients: rage quit. *Apparently the term is usually used in the context of video games, but I think it sums up what many people experience on diets. They lose their way, and they quit in a state of rage toward the book or person who suggested yet another unsustainable diet. And then they feel rage toward themselves. That's not going to happen anymore—because rage toward yourself is unacceptable! You deserve better than that.*

So, no more dieting in the usual sense. And yes, what you eat matters. In the next chapter, we'll talk about which foods will best help you achieve your goals. We are fully aware that simply *knowing* what to eat doesn't work if that's not what you're eating in real life—and we'll help you with that, too.

Janice—Many scientists who have studied weight loss claim that the diet most likely to work is the diet you're most likely to stay with. Well, I'm not so sure I agree with that—at least, not entirely. The goal is not merely to get thinner. Don't you also want to feel healthy and vibrant and energetic? Sure, you can lose weight by eating nothing more than a cupcake a day washed down with diet soda—but you'll feel awful, and your body won't thank you one bit.

Journalist Michael Pollan puts it best when he sums up how we should eat: "Eat food. Mostly plants. Not too much."[1] In other words, **eat real food**.

It couldn't be simpler. So, what's the problem? Why aren't people doing this? Why do Americans keep getting heavier and heavier? We're going to discuss the reasons in more depth, but here are some of the major ones:

- "Desirable," unhealthy processed foods are everywhere. You can find delicious junk filled with sugar, fat, and salt wherever you turn.

- Portion control is out of control. We are eating too much (at least too much processed food).
- Sugar-sweetened drinks add empty calories and subtract from healthy eating. Processed food often already contains added sugar, but sugary drinks are their own special brand of terrible.
- Dining out can be a booby trap of temptation. Restaurant portions tend to be huge, and a lot of the food in restaurants is unhealthy.
- A sedentary lifestyle has become the norm. Most Americans simply aren't physically active enough.

The "modern" Western diet has caught up with all of us. The vast quantities of processed foods that so many people consume in large quantities are unhealthy for them and their children. It's not just that people who eat this way are dying earlier than they should—it's that they are living with more disease, more medication, less energy, and less sense of well-being.

A study of American men and women found that if they make no changes in how they eat, they gain between one and three pounds per year.[2] By the way, in that study, foods associated with the greatest weight gain were potato chips, potatoes, sugary drinks, and red meat. Foods associated with weight loss, on the other hand, were vegetables, whole grains, fruits, nuts, and yogurt. Many other studies have found similar results.[3]

Candyland

Why do people have such a difficult time eating in a healthier way? It's particularly challenging for those who were not exposed to healthy eating as children. There is no easy fix for this because convenient, delicious, unhealthy, cheap food is everywhere, and it's tantalizing. As the authors of the book *The Evolution of Obesity* put it, "We evolved on the savannahs of Africa; we now live in Candyland."[4]

Food companies bear at least a good part of the responsibility for this "Candyland" phenomenon and the perpetuation of our country's obesity crisis. Recently, documents from the 1960s were uncovered revealing that the sugar industry paid eminent scientists to review only studies that minimized the role of sugar in heart disease and maximized the damaging effects of fat.[5] Those "findings" were then published in a prestigious medical journal. After that, for decades, people ate low-fat and non-fat processed foods that were allegedly healthier because of their lowered fat content. And what made these foods palatable? The answer is sugar, particularly in the form of high-fructose corn syrup,[6] which was added to the food.

In Chapter 6, we'll be talking about the potentially addictive power of sugar. Food companies know this and take advantage of it. In his book *Sugar, Salt, Fat*, investigative journalist Michael Moss explains how the food industry capitalizes on the "Bliss Point"—that allegedly magical place of just the perfect amount of sugar (often with added salt and fat) to make food completely irresistible.[7] The advertisement for potato chips where the tagline is "Bet you can't eat just one!" is no joke. As the authors of one study put it, "If certain foods are addictive, this may partially explain the difficulty people experience in achieving sustainable weight loss . . . Ubiquitous food advertising and the availability of inexpensive palatable foods may make it extremely difficult to adhere to healthier food choices because the omnipresent food cues trigger the reward system."[8] The "addictive" potential of some processed foods is no accident.

In his book *The End of Overeating*, former FDA Commissioner Dr. David A. Kessler acknowledges how food stimulates the brain and how food corporations have exploited this: "Over the last three decades, modern global food companies have taken full advantage of this weakness of human biology, putting high-fat, high-sugar, and high-salt foods within constant, immediate reach . . . the only surprise may be that some people have managed to resist."[9] No wonder we had to write this book!

Jae—Financial concerns also make weight loss in this day and age an uphill battle. In a country where you can get a double cheeseburger and McChicken for two dollars and fifty cents, while a small box of fresh baby bella mushrooms is three dollars, the ability to eat healthy and natural foods can depend on a person's socioeconomic status.

Food industry scientists are paid not to research natural, healthy foods, but rather to develop processed foods that taste so good that people crave them. The industry then hires both marketing experts to advertise directly to children and adults and lobbyists to stop efforts to tax sugary drinks or to stop direct advertising to children.[10] Is this a conspiracy? Is the food industry trying to make us fat with its "obesogenic marketing"?[11] In a way, the answer is no. The food industry is simply that—an industry, a business that must compete in our economy by employing strategies that are part of a free enterprise system. But there are serious, damaging consequences to this profit-driven system. Luckily, the bottom-line is that you're an adult. You get to decide what to eat. If you choose to eat unhealthy processed food regularly or occasionally, that's up to you. But it's different with kids. They cannot make the same considered decisions that adults supposedly can. The food industry uses television and internet commercials, mascots, video games, and promotional products to directly advertise to kids.

Janice—I accept that the food industry is a business that has responsibilities to its stockholders. But aren't there other stakeholders, too? At the very least, is there no responsibility to our country's children?

But do not despair that there is no possible way to resist all these temptations! The good news is there are concrete and specific actions you can take to lessen the influence of ever-present unhealthy processed foods. It's not impossible—the two of us are living proof! It's time, then, to talk about precisely what to eat and how to eat in a way that is healthy, satisfying, and sustainable for the rest of your life.

Janice—In doing research for this book, I have read several hundred scientific and medical journal articles. I've learned three major things:

1. Scientists and doctors are very confused about food and nutrients.
2. Vegetables and fruits are really, really good for us.
3. Processed foods are not.

What does healthy eating mean? It's quite simple, really. Here are the foods we recommend as the basis for what to eat:

- Vegetables
- Fruits
- Whole grains
- Lean protein
- Certain plant-based fats

Instead of eating fresh, high-fiber, nutrient-dense, minimally processed foods, so many people tend to eat garbage and then take vitamin supplements in order to keep "healthy." Do not be deceived: the vitamins in supplements are *not* the same as the vitamins in food. For reasons that are not fully understood, most of the vitamins contained in supplements have far fewer benefits than those contained in food.[12]

Science You Can Use! Glycemic Index & Glycemic Load

The word *carbohydrates* refers to so many different kinds of food that the term is confusing and even misleading. Even terms like *good carbs* and *bad carbs* are problematic because they give labels to foods that may not deserve them. A much more useful way to categorize carbohydrates in terms of their health effects on the body is to consider glycemic index and glycemic load. Stay with us here.

The glycemic index (GI) ranks carbohydrates according to how much they raise blood sugar levels after you eat them. Foods with a high GI are quickly digested and cause large fluctuations in blood sugar levels. High GI foods will satisfy your hunger more quickly, but they also leave you with an "energy crash" sooner—causing you to eat more to compensate. Low-GI foods, on the other hand, are digested more slowly. This means blood levels of glucose and insulin rise slowly and stay more stable. And that's a good thing—for both your health and your level of hunger.

While, the **glycemic index** measures how much a given food affects blood glucose, **glycemic load** takes into account the total amount of food that is eaten. In other words, one potato is associated with a certain glycemic index, and three potatoes triples the glycemic load.

What's the big deal about low-glycemic-load diets? Twenty-five years of data has shown that there is greater weight loss associated with low-glycemic-load diets.[13,14] One of the reasons for this is low-glycemic-load diets help to control appetite and delay hunger.[15]

Even when there is equal weight loss among different diets, low-glycemic-load diets are much better at preventing diabetes, heart disease, and stroke. [16, 17, 18] On the other hand, high-glycemic-index refined carbohydrates, such as the sugar and flour in processed foods, are actually an independent risk factor for disease. It's more than just a simple matter of how many calories you eat and how much you weigh; instead, it's a matter of eating foods that will leave you feeling better, living longer, and needing less medication to treat preventable diseases. Every medication has side effects and costs money, so wouldn't you love to need less of it? And let's not forget that being in good health to begin with is much, much better than trying to medicate yourself back from poor health. As one researcher put it: "Dietary carbohydrate restriction reliably reduces high blood glucose . . . and leads to the reduction or elimination of medication. It has never shown side effects comparable with those seen in many drugs."[19]

More Science: Your Brain Wants Good Food

There's a wonderful little structure in the brain called the hippocampus. The job of the hippocampus has to do with learning, memory, and mood regulation. Processed foods, stress, and chronic inflammation decrease new growth of nerve cells in the hippocampus. Healthy foods, conversely, contain chemicals (especially omega-3 fatty acids, flavonoids, polyphenols, and antioxidants) that make the hippocampus very happy.[20]

The Intestinal Microbiome: You Really Are What You Eat!

You have more microorganisms inhabiting your body than you have your own cells. While that may sound a bit like something out of *Alien*, it's not—it's essential for life. A hundred trillion bacteria in the gastrointestinal tract, along with some viruses and fungi, form what is referred to as the *gut microbiota* or *microbiome*. And what you eat is the major determinant of which microbes decide to take up residence in your intestines.[21]

"So what?" you might ask. Here's what: the amount, type, and diversity of these bacteria actually play a large role in how easily you gain or lose weight.[22, 23] That may sound like science fiction, but it's true! The types of bacteria that live in your intestine help determine not just your intestinal function, but also the health of your heart and liver, as well as your immune, respiratory, and metabolic systems.[24, 25] These bacteria help determine how you respond to medications, and the microbiome affects how your nervous system works to affect brain function, mood, and behavior.[26] So, you see, the effect of the intestinal microbiome reaches far beyond the intestine to influence other parts of the body's physical and mental functions.[27]

Research clearly shows that the constituents of the gut microbiome are not one bit happy about the typical Western diet,[28] meaning a diet containing lots of animal fats, processed foods, and refined sugar. Human intestines that are fed a typical Western diet have a microbiome that is less varied (which is a bad thing) and is functionally inferior to that of people who eat a diet rich in vegetables, fruits, and whole grains.[29, 30] This unhealthy microbiome is strongly correlated with not just intestinal diseases, such as irritable bowel syndrome, and inflammatory bowel diseases, such as Crohn's disease and ulcerative colitis, but also with metabolic syndrome, diabetes, heart disease, allergies, autoimmune illnesses, asthma, diabetes, and some cancers—all of which are related to chronic low-grade systemic inflammation.[31, 32]

Timing is Everything: The Night Kitchen

It's not just *what* you eat, but *when* you eat it. This is at least partially related to the microbiome, as well as to the body's hormones, all of which respond to daily circadian rhythms, those twenty-four-hour cycles that affect the body's functions.[33] Insulin levels, in particular, are lower at night. Your body simply doesn't metabolize glucose as well later in the day—and this increases your risk for obesity, diabetes, and heart disease, even if the overall number of calories you consume hasn't increased.[34] Other hormones are affected as well, which may partially explain why people who eat more at night may be at increased risk for cancer, particularly breast cancer.[35]

Another problem with eating at night is that it is associated with poorer sleep quality,[36] which, as we'll discuss in Chapter 16, threatens physical and mental health, emotional well-being, and weight control. Finally, people who eat later at night tend to consume more calories than people who ingest most of their calories earlier in the day.[37] That comes as no surprise. Let's face it: no one craves broccoli at eleven o'clock at night.

Fasting—Super or Stupid?

Janice—While there's a lot of talk out there about the supposed health and weight loss benefits of fasting, there's not a whole lot of scientific information. Having said that, I do think there's enough solid information about three types of fasting for me to make some recommendations.

1. Alternate-Day Fasting

In this model, you eat zero calories every other day. Then, on alternate days, there's no restriction on calories. The biggest problem with this plan is a simple one: *hunger.* Some people are really hungry on fast days (big surprise, right?), and this does not always decrease with time.[38] This hunger state is bound to lead to an unsustainable feeling of deprivation. What is more, this strategy is associated with only mild weight loss and no improvement in glucose metabolism.[39] And here's the kicker: your mood may worsen with alternate-day fasting.[40]

Janice's Verdict: Pretty Stupid

2. Intermittent Modified Fasting

This regimen refers to decreasing caloric intake on fasting days, usually to about 25 percent that of non-fasting days. There do not seem to be any health or weight loss benefits greater than with general caloric restriction.[41] Also, persistent hunger may be a problem with this regimen, too.

Janice's Verdict: Why Bother?

3. Time-Restricted Eating

Time-restricted eating refers to avoiding food later at night or closer to bedtime, which we discussed in detail above.

Janice's Verdict: Super!

The Effect is Profound

When people make a switch to a healthier diet with less meat and fewer processed foods, they lose abdominal fat and lower their risk of getting metabolic syndrome and type 2 diabetes.[42] This is at least partly because of the change in the microbiome. What is more, this change can happen quickly, even within a matter of days.[43]

Changing to a healthier, less processed, more plant-based diet brings about the same dramatic, rapid changes in the intestines of children, as well. Breastfeeding is good for an infant's microbiome.[44] However, by the time children are three years old, even if they were breastfed as babies, they'll have the same intestinal bacteria makeup as adults. This provides even more proof that what we feed children really matters and is crucial to their health and development.[45]

What Diet is Best for a Healthy Microbiome?

The answer is pretty simple: more plant-based foods and fewer processed foods and meat. The healthy, natural chemicals in fruits and vegetables, along with the fiber in non-animal foods, are the best sources of the ingredients you need for a robust intestinal microbiome.[46]

There's an exception to the non-processed, plant-based recommendation. Bacteria-fermented foods such as yogurt is an abundant source of probiotics, which are the bacteria that are specifically healthy for the intestine. Which brings us to our next, brief science lesson.

Probiotics & Prebiotics

Probiotics, whether in foods or supplements, contain live organisms that supply your intestine with healthy microbes. Probiotic foods include kefir, yogurt, sauerkraut, kimchi, and kombucha (a brilliant alternative to soda).

Prebiotics, on the other hand, are not organisms, but rather indigestible plant fibers from many fruits and vegetables, as well as whole grains that serve as a food source for the intestinal bacteria themselves.[47]

Why Not Just Take Probiotic & Prebiotic Supplements?

Probiotic and prebiotic supplements may have value. They do not seem to have significant risks. The problem with recommending them is that, at the time of this publication, there aren't standards to ensure that what is inside the bottle is what the outside of the bottle says there is, both in content and amount.

Even if the species, strains, and dosages are specified, there are currently no product purity or labeling standards for probiotics to ensure that what is listed on the probiotic supplement label is actually what is in the bottle.[48, 49] What is more, there's a lot of variation with regard to how individual people respond to individual probiotics.[50]

Final Thought

Please don't feel bad about yourself based on what you eat. Give up the guilt and the shame, both of which are useless and destructive. But *do* think about what a gift you're giving to yourself in terms of physical, mental, and emotional health when you reach for that apple.

Trust your gut, literally. That is, if you eat the right stuff. Now, let's talk more about this *right stuff.*

CHAPTER 5

Foods That Love You Back

> When people go on crazy diets and feel miserable, not only do they gain the weight back, but they also end up weighing more than they did—as a survival strategy to avoid starvation.

It's probably clear to you by now that this is not a conventional diet book; that's why it's taken us until Chapter 5 to get around to recommending what foods you should eat. We want to help you lose excess weight in a way that will allow you to feel more alive and vital and to provide you with strategies to make that happen permanently. The health rewards you will reap from eating a diet of real foods are incredible. In this chapter, we'll go into the details about these wonderful foods. Read on.

Vegetables: Your New Best Friend

We firmly believe that if you don't eat a lot of vegetables, you simply cannot lose weight in a healthy way or eat enough food to keep you from a state of hunger and deprivation. Humans are hardwired to be intolerant of deprivation; it's a survival thing. That's why when people go on crazy diets and feel miserable, not only do they gain the weight back, but they also end up weighing more than they did—as a survival strategy to avoid starvation. Vegetables are your key to being able to eat a lot of food with fantastic health benefits and without the calories.

A clarification: vegetables, in the context of this book, refer to non-starchy vegetables. Starchy vegetables include potatoes, corn, and peas; and these vegetables have a relatively high glycemic index. Furthermore, they are actually associated with weight gain, not loss.[1]

Eating five or more servings a day of fruits and vegetables (especially vegetables) is strongly associated with a longer life span.[2] And it's not just longer—it's better! It's longer life where you'll have the greater chance of feeling good and moving freely.

We need to give a special shout-out to cruciferous vegetables, such as broccoli, cauliflower, Brussels sprouts, kale, cabbage, and bok choy. Cruciferous vegetables are the healthiest of the healthy foods you can eat. They contain chemicals that fight many, many types of cancers,[3, 4, 5, 6] they contain a ton of fiber, and they last a relatively long time in your refrigerator. You can roast them, stir-fry them, steam them, grill them, or even eat them raw—we'll offer you several recipes in our recipe section (page 265).

Store-bought vegetables and fruits that are already cut up cost more and probably aren't as fresh—but if that's what it takes for you to eat them, then do it! It's certainly better than not eating them at all because you're too pressed for time or you find that chopping is too much of a hassle. Moreover, whatever you pay for this "luxury" costs a lot less than what you would have to pay for medications to treat various health conditions down the road.

Be curious and have fun trying new and varied vegetables and fruits. Instead of just walking past unfamiliar ones, check out what's available in your market (especially what's seasonal and local). You can always look up recipes that use those foods and see what appeals to you. Perhaps you'll have a brand-new vegetable on your shopping list and a new recipe to try. What's the worst that can happen? You won't like it, and you'll try something else. If you feel timid about cooking something new, then make an effort to sample an unfamiliar dish at a restaurant. Try something from the vegetarian section of the menu, or go to a restaurant that specializes in vegetarian cooking.

Janice—This doesn't apply just to vegetables. Be open to new eating experiences. For a long time, I always refused to eat tofu; I insisted it tasted like phlegm. Then Jae made me her marinated sautéed tofu (it's in our recipe section on page 302) and now I'm a true believer! Play with seasonings and spices, new foods, and new ways of preparing old ones.

Fruits: Sweetness without Deprivation

Yes, fruits do have sugars in them, but what makes them different from sugar-laden processed foods, particularly when high-fructose corn syrup is an ingredient, is that the fructose in fruit comes along with fiber, which slows down the absorption of sugar and decreases the spike in blood glucose after eating. This is particularly important for people with diabetes,[7] but it also means you won't get hungry again so soon after eating.

Fruits contain lots of other nutrients as well, meaning that they are not only delicious, but also filling and healthy. Many people find that once they've gone for a long time without refined sugar, fruit actually does satisfy their "sweet tooth." Despite the sugar content, eating fruit is actually associated with weight *loss;* whereas weight *gain* is the result of comparable refined sugar intake. You're never going to reach an unhappy weight from eating too many apples! If you're diabetic, do eat more fruits that have a lower glycemic index, such as berries, citrus fruits, apples, and pears.

Jae—*Try freezing fruit! A friend introduced me to frozen raspberries, which seriously taste like sorbet. I grew up in Michigan blueberry farm country—we would pick buckets of them during the summer. My mom would wash them, let them air dry (this is important—it reduces crinkling and freezer burn), and then freeze them. She put them over ice cream then, but now I use them as a snack or to blend into smoothies or add on the top of yogurt.*

Speaking of smoothies, they're a great way to introduce fruits and vegetables into your diet. It's really easy to blend in healthy foods like spinach, flax or chia seeds, or beets without changing the flavor of the smoothie, which already has delicious fruits and/or kefir or yogurt (we've got a recipe for you on page 305). A word of caution: do not confuse smoothies with juicing. Juicing both removes the fiber (which is what helps you stay fuller for longer) from the fruit and concentrates the sugars.

Fiber: A Magical Component

Fiber-rich foods are treasures. In addition to vegetables and fruits, foods high in fiber include whole grains (such as brown rice, wild rice, oatmeal, quinoa, barley, and bulgur), beans, legumes, nuts, and seeds. Fiber-rich diets are associated with a lower risk of cardiovascular disease,[8] certain cancers,[9] and many inflammation-associated conditions such as diabetes and heart disease.[10, 11]

Jae—*I've had quite the journey with vegetables—well, high-fiber, healthy foods more generally. Until after my freshman year of college, I ate mostly convenient and fast food. The summer I lived with vegetarians, though, I tried new foods that my roommates prepared. In the end, I learned to love all kinds of foods that I never would have given a chance before.*

Now I buy vegetables all the time, paying attention to which ones are in season. Usually I roast them or steam them. I love to play with different seasonings and hot sauce.

Since that time, I've added fish and poultry back into my diet, but learning to eat varied and copious amounts of vegetables was integral in changing my lifestyle and food preferences. I still eat very little animal meat—I get most of my protein from chickpeas, black beans, and yogurt.

A common group of high-fiber foods are legumes, which consist of foods like beans, nuts, peas, and lentils. We can't say enough about the humble bean. Beans are incredible—they are cheap, they keep for a really long time, they're loaded with protein and fiber, and they're really, really filling!

There are so many types of beans, and we recommend experimenting with different types and using them in various ways—try them in salads and soups, for example. Dried beans are cheaper, but canned beans are just as fine and awfully convenient. Just check the label and make sure you're getting plain old beans and not "traditional" baked beans with added sugar, sodium, and all kinds of junk.

A common worry for people who are increasing the amount of legumes in their diet (which includes beans) is intestinal gas. If you find that it's a problem, start out by eating fewer beans until your intestinal tract adjusts. Here's another trick: soak dried beans for a longer time and change the water every so often—you'll have much less gas.

Many healthy high-fiber foods, such as nuts, legumes, and whole grains, are relatively high in calories; but because they are so filling, whole grains (but *not* refined grains such as white bread, white rice, white or corn tortillas, and pasta) are associated with loss of both weight and abdominal fat.[12]

Pulses (dried peas, beans, and lentils) are inexpensive, nutrient-packed, and have one of the lowest carbon footprints of any food. They are full of protein and rich in fiber, iron, folate, and potassium.

Janice—Doctors (including me, at one time) would tell patients that losing weight was "a simple equation—calories in need to be less than calories out." Well, not only is that useless "advice," but it turns out that it's not even true! The type *of calories can make a difference. People lose more weight when they eat a diet that's higher in fat than when they eat the same number of calories in a diet that's higher in (high-glycemic-index) carbohydrates.*[13] *Why is that? It's because it takes more energy to burn certain foods (mainly high-fiber foods) than others, which is precisely what we want to do in order to lose more weight.*

Fats: Have We All Gotten the Wrong Advice?

As we mentioned earlier, for several decades now, "thanks" largely to processed foods, the obesity rate in this country has continued to rise, even as people have been eating more fat-free and low-fat foods. That's because when people go on low-fat diets, they tend to get hungrier and to increase their consumption of refined carbohydrates, especially sugar.[14] Fat may have been unfairly maligned all this time as the bad guy.[15, 16]

There are many different kinds of fats, some of which actually are terrible, and some of which belong in everyone's diet. The truly Bad Fat is the group of manufactured **trans fats,** which are added to foods as a way to extend shelf life.[17] These trans fats should be avoided altogether.[18]

Saturated fats are found in animal foods, primarily meat and dairy products, as well as in coconut products. Current thinking is that they may not significantly contribute to the risk of heart disease.[19] Even full-fat dairy is getting more recognition due to its ability to prevent weight gain (because it is more "filling" than low-fat or non-fat options), and, as a result, prevent diabetes and heart disease.[20]

There is a third major group of fats: **unsaturated fats**. These are actually great for us. There is a lower risk of dying earlier when saturated fats in the diet are replaced by polyunsaturated fats,[21] which are abundant in walnuts, flax seeds, and fatty fish, such as salmon, mackerel, and sardines. Monounsaturated fats, found in plant foods such as olive oil (especially extra-virgin olive oil), nuts, and avocados are also extremely healthy.[22]

Fish: A Friend to Your Brain and Your Body

Eating fish has considerable health benefits for most people. We recommend that you eat plenty of it, ideally twice a week.[23] There's even good evidence that people who eat greater quantities of oily fish are less likely to suffer cognitive decline and even Alzheimer's disease.[24]

However, due to the widespread presence of pesticides and heavy metals like mercury, young children and pregnant or breastfeeding women need to limit ingestion of certain fish, such as mackerel, albacore tuna, orange roughy, and swordfish.[25, 26] For these people, fish oil and other DHA supplements may make sense. However, note that, a recent analysis of studies involving thousands of people with heart disease showed that fish oil supplements are of little benefit,[27] and real fish is the way to go. The Environmental Protection Agency updates fish safety concerns and is a good source for news and recommendations for which kinds of fish are safest to consume. For the rest of us, fish like wild salmon that are high in omega-3 fatty acids are a fantastic source of nutrients.

Don't be afraid of frozen fish. In fact, unless you live next to a dock, it may be fresher than "fresh" fish. Frozen fish is often flash frozen on the boat right where it was caught. Plus, you can stock up on it when it's on sale.

Red Meat: A Red Flag

It's time to stop eating so much meat. A lot of research is looking into the effects of diets high in meat content, especially red meat. If you choose not to give up meat completely, then eat it less frequently and in smaller quantities. It's time for everyone to start thinking of meat as a side dish.

Numerous studies have shown that higher intake of red and processed meat (such as cold cuts and hot dogs) is associated with increased mortality, particularly from heart disease and cancer.[28, 29] Substituting as little as one serving per day typically reserved for meat with other sources of protein, such as fish, beans, legumes, nuts, poultry, and whole grains, lowers the mortality risk by as much as nearly 20 percent.[30]

Grass-fed meat, as well as meat from non-domesticated animals, however, is another matter. Grass-fed meat is from animals that are allowed to graze in pastures. Not only is grass-fed beef a more humane[31] and sustainable way to obtain beef, but it is also higher in healthy omega-3 fatty acids and B vitamins than the meat from cows who get a typical corn-and-soy-based feed. Yes, grass-fed meat is more expensive, but if you eat meat less often and in smaller quantities (because of all the vegetables and grains you're eating), then the cost can be less prohibitive.

Poultry & Eggs: A Chicken in Every Pot?

Poultry is kind of a neutral food. While it doesn't increase the risk of heart disease and breast cancer the way red meat does, it also doesn't reduce the risk the way plant-based proteins do.[32]

There is still much uncertainty about eggs.[33] While scientists no longer consider dietary cholesterol to be the main contributor to elevated cholesterol in the body, there's still a recommendation that people with elevated risk for heart disease limit their consumption of eggs and have instead a diet rich in lipid-lowering properties; that is, a diet rich in vegetables, fruits, whole grains, and fish.

Bread: Is It a Problem? Well, That Depends

Whole grain bread has a higher fiber content, which means it causes greater satiety and a more favorable shift in the intestinal bacteria compared to white bread. This is probably why it has been found that whole grain bread is not associated with weight gain, whereas white bread is.[34]

It's not quite that simple, though. The way in which bread is labeled can be extremely misleading. For example, you might find a loaf of bread advertised as "wheat bread" and think that sounds a lot like whole-wheat or whole-grain bread. But "wheat bread" is just bread! And many bread manufacturers add sugar to make it taste better and caramel coloring to make it look whole-grainier. Ridiculous.

Do consider delicious, healthy, even gluten-free versions of bread. For example, socca, or farinata, a French or Italian bread made with chickpea flour, is sensational and easy to make.

Dairy: Lots of Confusion

There's a lack of certainty regarding whole-fat dairy.[35] There have been suggestions that whole-fat milk is satisfying enough to cause people to consume fewer calories from other foods, especially processed carbohydrates. This may be true for children and adolescents as well.[36, 37]

Higher-fat milk is more filling, but lower-fat milk has less saturated fat. So, which is better? The answer depends on what else you eat.[38] For example, children are better off eating one cookie along with a glass of full-fat milk, rather than eating two cookies with a glass of non-fat milk—the fat in the milk is a lot healthier than the processed sugary stuff that's in the cookie. Bottom line: if you drink a glass of non-fat or low-fat milk and don't need to eat anything else until your next meal, that's great. But if you eat six cookies with a glass of skim milk in order to feel satisfied, you'd be much better off eating less cookies with the whole (full-fat) milk.

Water, Water Everywhere

We love water, and we drink plenty of it. The typical recommendation, admittedly based on limited data,[39] is to drink eight 8-ounce glasses of water a day. You don't want to be thirsty or dehydrated. So, yes, drink your water—but no, you are not a fish. Forcing yourself to drink water all day all the time is unnecessary. *However*, drinking 16 ounces of water an hour before a meal? Now that's a great idea—start filling up that belly! There is actual evidence[40] that this is a successful strategy for losing weight and for maintaining weight loss.

Alcohol: What About It?

For most of us, drinking a moderate amount of alcohol (one drink a day for women and two drinks a day for men) is fine—especially if it's red wine, which has specific health benefits.[41] High alcohol consumption, on the other hand, in addition to being toxic to the brain and liver, is related to an increased risk of cancer and death.[42, 43] Also, the pattern of drinking matters: the health benefits of having one drink a day do not apply to drinking seven drinks once a week.[44]

Alcohol can lead to weight gain[45] in several ways:

- You're drinking a lot of calories.
- If you're intoxicated, you're not functioning at your highest cognitive level; as a result, you're more likely to make poor eating and drinking choices.[46]
- Alcohol causes the level of blood sugar to drop; and, as a consequence, you may crave unhealthy carbohydrates.

Salt Is Not a Food That Loves You Back

Salt will definitely cause health problems if you have hypertension. However, even if you have normal blood pressure, while eating salt won't raise your pressure, it may still be bad news for your blood vessels.[47] What's more, adding salt to fatty food (think steak) increases the amount of that unhealthy food you want to eat.[48]

The good news is that if you decrease the amount of food you put salt on and the amount of salty foods you eat (check labels!), you will be pleasantly surprised at how quickly your taste buds will adjust to wanting your food to be less salty. In the meantime, you can still get wild and crazy with spices!

We're Not Done Yet

Throughout this book, we've stressed the physical and emotional toll that refined sugar exacts on you. Sugar, we're afraid, "deserves" its own chapter. Let's get to it.

STEP THREE:

Eat What You Want. But What Do You *Want?*

CHAPTER 6

Sugar—the Ultimate Comfort Food or the Work of the Devil?

The brain simply doesn't register "fullness" from sugar in drinks.

What's the answer to that question? You know it by now, of course: it's both. Here's the full story.

Janice—First, I have a very personal story to tell you. I am the daughter of a candy manufacturer. No, the irony of that is not lost on me. My father made candy canes and came home from work smelling like peppermint every day—it was great. I never objected to his portrayal of sugar as the feel-good elixir of life, but I must say that I'm glad he's not alive to read this book.

Witness for the Prosecution

We admit that we trash-talk sugar throughout this book, and there are several reasons for this. Here are a few:

- Delicious processed foods that are rich in sugar are a major dietary contributor to obesity.
- Foods high in sugar "feed" the brain's reward centers, much like the way opiates do.
- As a result, people crave—and may even show signs of being addicted to—these foods.
- On the other hand, the sugar in fruit, fructose, is absorbed slowly into the body because of all the fiber that's in fruit. Fruit does not contribute to obesity or obesity-related diseases.

In the author's note of Gary Taubes's powerful book, *The Case Against Sugar*,[1] he writes, "The purpose of this book is to present the case against sugar . . . as the principal cause of the chronic diseases that are most likely to kill us . . . in the twenty-first century. . . . If this were a criminal case, *The Case Against Sugar* would be the argument for the prosecution." It's a strong case.

Sugar in Drinks: It Only Gets Worse

Do you like to start your day with a glass of orange juice with your breakfast? Or have a bottle of soda with lunch? Here's an astonishing fact: when you eat *solid* sugary food, eventually your brain says, "Enough already!" But not so with liquids. The brain simply doesn't register "fullness" from sugar in drinks.[2] This means that when you have a sugary beverage, you'll still want to eat the same amount of food as if you hadn't had that drink. To make matters worse, this effect seems to be even more pronounced in children and adolescents.[3]

Not only that, sugar-based drinks do not quench thirst as well as water.[4] This means you need to drink more of them—and therefore ingest even more calories—in order to feel that you've quenched your thirst.[5] It's no wonder that sugar-sweetened beverages, the number one source of added sugar in Americans' diet, are the *single biggest dietary culprit in long-term weight gain.*[6]

Soda. Gulp.

Why is soda so dreadful? We've talked about how when you eat fruit, the body gets a pretty small "dose" of fructose.[7] On the other hand, high fructose corn syrup (HFCS), which is the form of fructose in soda (as well as many processed foods), is *not* absorbed slowly the way the fructose in fruit is. HFCS overloads the poor liver with an amazingly large amount of free fructose,[8] which then goes on to increase fat production and decrease the effectiveness of insulin in the body.

Soda and other sugar-sweetened beverages directly contribute to the prevalence of obesity, diabetes, heart disease, cavities in teeth, and possibly, in the case of some sodas, osteoporosis.[9] Almost two-thirds of children and adolescents in this country have at least one soda a day, and it is a major contributor to obesity in childhood and later in life.[10, 11]

Janice—*This is just my opinion, but it's one based on what I've learned from scientists who are a whole lot smarter than I am: I don't think there's a good reason to have sugary soda in the house. Ever. Especially if you have kids. It's worth negotiating forcefully on that subject.*

The Soda Industry Won't Go Down without a Fight

Perhaps not surprisingly, the soda industry has funded studies that somehow "prove" that sugar-sweetened beverages do not cause weight gain and its health consequences.[12] Worse still, the major soda companies have lobbied against numerous public health bills that were intended to reduce soda consumption or improve nutrition[13] and furthermore have developed marketing strategies specifically directed to children.[14] Recently, in Philadelphia where the mayor proposed a soda tax,[15] citizens were deluged with commercials opposing the proposed "beverage tax" that was "causing pain to working families." Oh, come on now.

How about Fruit Juice?

Fruit juice is better than soda, but that's about the best we can say for it. Following a policy statement from the American Academy of Pediatrics in 2017, even pediatricians now recommend against letting children drink fruit juice freely.[16] Compared with whole fruit, juice contains concentrated sugar and none of the fiber. Fruit juice is a major contributor to childhood obesity, as well as tooth decay.[17] Having said that, at least fruit juice has vitamins and healthy phytochemicals—soda doesn't. Just don't drink a lot of juice or give kids much of it at all. Give them water with an apple instead of apple juice.

Diet Drinks: Are You Kidding Yourself?

Sorry, diet soda is not the answer. It doesn't do as much damage to your health and weight as regular soda, but that's faint praise. For one thing, people lose more weight when they drink water than when they drink artificially sweetened drinks.[18] This may be because artificial sweeteners do not diminish the continued craving for sugary food.[19, 20] What's the solution? Treat yourself to a bowl of strawberries and a cup of tea.

Also, while there aren't good studies comparing the specific metabolic effects of different sweeteners,[21] they do change the intestinal microbiome in a way that may lead to more glucose intolerance[22] and diabetes. To make matters worse, "artificially sweetened soft drink consumption has been associated with a higher risk of stroke and dementia."[23]

Jae—I stopped drinking pop a few years ago, and this change has made me feel so much better. I save so much money, and I know I'm doing something good for my body. After all this time not drinking pop, I no longer crave, want, or even like pop. I tried it the other week and it tasted so disgusting.

Janice—I finally gave up my Diet Coke habit. But every so often, I have some; and you know what? I still love it. Too bad, Janice—get over it.

Let's end this chapter on an upbeat note: making a single healthy change in your diet, like giving up these drinks, will not only add to your overall health, but also motivate you to make other healthy changes.[24] Ditch the soda.

CHAPTER 7

What's Comfort? What's Deprivation? Are You Sure?

"Eating your feelings" started as a
way to comfort and protect yourself,
but it has now become destructive.

Janice—*I'm at a breakfast meeting at work. I help myself to fruit and yogurt—but then I see those muffins, and they look totally amazing. I know that "muffin" is a breakfast euphemism for "cake"—especially the one with the sugary crumb topping. Don't I deserve at least a little reward for having to sit through this long meeting? Why should I have to deprive myself? I could take a muffin and have just one bite now and then another bite after lunch and then finish it for an afternoon snack. And then just have steamed broccoli for dinner. That's my plan.*

There's a problem with this so-called plan. In fact, there are several problems. First of all, I will have finished the whole muffin before the end of the meeting. Second, never in a million years am I going to eat nothing more than steamed broccoli for dinner. I know this. Once that muffin catches my eye and I allow myself to even consider eating it, I'm in trouble. The muffin is clouding my thinking with its promise of sweet crumbly bliss. And here's the really big problem: because of avoiding "deprivation" and seemingly "rewarding" myself, I will feel disgusted with myself thirty seconds later, when I have devoured the entire muffin. I will begin an inner dialogue that may last for the rest of the day, reminding myself that I am a complete failure and that I am seriously lacking self-discipline and willpower. This is a reward? And by the way, this inner dialogue will keep me from having the slightest idea of what is going on in the meeting!

Does this sound familiar? If you're on a diet and feel deprived, the chance of failure is pretty close to one hundred percent. We humans find deprivation to be intolerable. Losing weight using a conventional diet (i.e., one that tells you what you can eat, what you cannot eat, and how much you can eat) creates a feeling of deprivation. People who lose weight in such a scenario almost always gain the weight back. Not only that, but they also usually gain more weight than they had lost and end up weighing even more than when they had started. This whole spiral began because they wanted to avoid the feeling of deprivation. We imagine you know how this feels; most of us have been there—perhaps several times.

Here's how conventional diets work: to lose weight, you decide to cut out "comfort foods." Then you have a Really Bad Day, and you tell yourself you "deserve" to eat something comforting. And let's be honest, "comfort food" never refers to celery; instead, it is mostly about sugar or fat or salt—or all three. When you eat foods high in sugar, fat, or salt in order to feel better, you may find, as we both do, that you'll start feeling like a shark tasting blood—you just want more. So you eat more—maybe a lot more. And you know what? You *do* feel better for a few minutes. Calmer, less anxious. Maybe a little sleepy. But then what happens? We now present to you:

The Comfort Food Circle of Hell

- I want a cookie.
- I find the package of cookies that I'd supposedly hidden from myself.
- I eat a cookie.
- I want another cookie. Even more than the first one.
- I eat another cookie. And another.
- I feel better. Calmer. Soothed. Then numb. Then irritable.
- I realize what I have done and feel disgusted with myself.
- I feel like a failure.
- I want to feel better.
- I eat a cookie . . .

This cycle is the kind of pattern that ends in both physical and emotional misery. "Eating your feelings" started as a way to comfort and protect yourself, but it has now become destructive. There must be a better way. In fact, there is a better way. This better way does not mean giving up comfort or feeling chronically deprived. Rather, there needs to be a new type of satisfaction that no longer blurs the line between reward and punishment. There needs to be another paradigm shift:

Old Paradigm	New Paradigm
Why should I deprive myself of food that I love and that will comfort me?	Real deprivation is when I eat food that decreases my quality of life.
I eat my feelings to comfort and protect myself.	Taking care of my body, mentally and physically, comforts and protects me.
If I don't get to eat the foods that I love, that is just one more thing that's taken from me.	By eating in a healthy way, I'm not losing anything– I'm adding to my life and to my happiness.

Janice—*Eating in an unhealthy way is what deprivation now means to me. It is this new paradigm that makes it possible for me to make a conscious decision to walk past the muffin. I am not telling myself that I can't eat the muffin, but rather that I am choosing not to eat the muffin. That's a totally different feeling, and it has helped me dig out of that self-defeating (not to mention unappealing) quagmire of feeling self-pity because of my struggles with weight.*

Jae—*Even though I've lost 142 pounds, it's still hard for me to stop turning to food for comfort. It's something I work on every day. I honestly thought that achieving a healthy weight would make all of my problems go away. Of course, that didn't happen. But I keep working on this because I know that I'm a much happier and healthier person now. I feel proud and accomplished.*

Our message to you is simple: you can develop a good relationship with your body and become a healthier version of yourself. A healthier life does not mean you will never again have another chocolate chip cookie. It does not mean you will never have cake on your birthday, or eat pumpkin pie on Thanksgiving, or enjoy a burger and fries when you go out with your friends. Rather, it means you'll *choose* to make choices that will result in the reward of looking good, feeling good, and moving freely. This way, you're focusing on what you're *adding* to your life, not on what you're giving up. At some point, you may find that you are able to choose to have the occasional muffin, but you won't be hypnotized or controlled by it. And you won't have to hear your Evil Twin telling you that you're weak and pathetic.

Comfort *is* important to all of us, but the promise of comfort food is, ultimately, a false one. Making a considered, conscious choice is an essential paradigm shift in the process of moving away from a deprivation mindset. It will help you feel in charge and competent, as well as equipped to find true sources of comfort. Not only that, but as a result of this paradigm shift, you will still enjoy food without using it as an emotional crutch. If you fundamentally change your relationship with food, eating becomes even more enjoyable because it will no longer be associated with guilt and shame. You will be proud of yourself for eating in a way that will support your emotional and physical health. And we're going to talk about how that can happen.

Reframing Comfort & Discomfort

Remember that mean voice in your head, the Evil Twin, that won't go away without a fight? What do you say to that voice that promises you comfort through a cookie? Simply this: you know that the cookie's promise of comfort is short-lived and even deceitful—and that feeling disgusted with yourself causes profound *discomfort*.

That discomfort can now be replaced by the deep satisfaction of realizing that you really feel better about yourself, and that returning to your old self-destructive ways is not a choice you are willing to make. With more practice, you will develop the confidence to make these positive choices more easily—they will become a habit, just as destructive choices were a habit in the past. Of course, reaching the point of feeling this way is easier said than done—but that's what this book is for. We want to take this step by step alongside you. In fact, we devote the entire Chapter 13 to changing habits permanently.

Janice—*Ultimately, I've had to redefine what I want to eat. Yes, I still wish that I could eat unlimited amounts of chocolate, but I also wish that I were tall and graceful. I've had to let go of those wishes—and the reward has been so much richer than the chocolate.*

Jae—For such a long time, I used food in order to comfort and protect myself, as a defense mechanism against feeling out of control. Once I recognized that this was a problem and not a solution, I identified it as a challenge I wanted to take on. From there, I made the decision to change what I put in my body. It was then that the role was reversed—I was on the offensive now. It was a new game, and I was ready to create strategies and skills in order to be effective in this new role.

Don't Stress Out

The first step is to think about, write about, and then act upon your self-identified non-food sources of comfort. There is ample evidence that chronic stress is associated with obesity (no surprise there), and that managing stress and alleviating discomfort are vital pieces of the healthy living puzzle. We'll be talking about stress and eating in detail in Chapters 15 through 17. In the meantime, it's time for the next list.

List #4: Your Non-Food Sources of Comfort

Think about what calms you, soothes you, and helps you relax that isn't food.

Jae's list:
write in my journal or in my gratitude journal
go for a run
take deep breaths
take a hot shower
call or spend time with friends
learn something new
explore a new area of the city
watch a show on Netflix

Janice's list:
dig out weeds in the garden
read a novel
call a friend
listen to classical music
dance to rock music
take the dog for a walk
watch a baseball game while I needlepoint
have a cup of ginger tea

Please make this list. Think of new strategies and activities that will help turn the list into reality. Try yoga? Learn to meditate? Join a community garden? Get a walking buddy? Think outside the box! The box of cookies, that is.

It All Adds up—In a Good Way!

Finding a new path is easy—anyone can lose five pounds, or even much more. Staying on that path, on the other hand, is where most people lose their way. It's hard to completely overhaul your routine and lifestyle. No wonder there are countless diet books, "miracle" products, and television promotions. We do not in any way deny that making the changes we propose throughout this book will be a challenge. Negative thoughts and feelings are incredibly powerful and have been ingrained for years. Unhealthy eating habits that developed to protect against these thoughts and feelings are powerful and ingrained, too.

But we also know from what science tells us, as well as from our real-life experiences, that changes in thoughts and behaviors are possible. By consistently acknowledging the meaningful changes you make—even pride in your ongoing *effort* to make these changes—you will continue to feel motivated and confident in your ability to keep going on the new path you have defined for yourself.

This cumulative **positive reinforcement** can help shift your way of thinking about comfort in a meaningful, long-lasting way. Eating your feelings does *not* provide true comfort, but feeling good about yourself *does*. When you make this paradigm shift and recognize that feeling in control and shedding shame are fantastic rewards, you will no longer feel that you are depriving yourself. Rather, you're taking care of yourself.

Janice—For me, positive reinforcement means that every time I make a healthy food decision and every time I exercise, I congratulate myself. When I eat fruit instead of ice cream, or when I walk the dog instead of just opening the door to let him out in the yard, I remember to tell myself that my body is thanking me. I tell myself how proud I am. I say it out loud sometimes (but only when I'm alone, since I sound like I'm talking to an eight-year-old). I certainly recommend writing down successes—the apple instead of the apple pie, the stairs instead of the elevator, going for a walk with a friend instead of having a lunch date at a pizzeria—these are all successes. Writing them down is another way to give myself credit.

Jae—Consciously making the effort to congratulate myself is so hard to keep in mind consistently, but I know how motivating for me it is to celebrate every victory. I'm kicking ass! I'm succeeding. I'm improving my quality of life. I remember that with every good choice, I'm accomplishing what I once thought was impossible.

True comfort comes when your brain and body are in harmony resulting from an appreciation of who you are. There's no food for that. Instead, let's look elsewhere.

CHAPTER 8

Creating a Diet That Isn't a Diet

> By changing the foods you eat
> regularly, you can absolutely change
> what your future health looks like.

No More "Going on a Diet"

Promise yourself that you'll never "go on a diet" again. Instead, let's put together what you learned in Chapter 6 to develop an action plan for eating the foods that love you back.

The rules are incredibly simple:

- Eat *lots* of non-starchy vegetables, fruits, beans and legumes, nuts, fish, extra-virgin olive oil, whole grains, and fermented foods (such as kefir, yogurt, sauerkraut, miso, and even pickles).[1]
- Eat less of everything else.

That's it. We're done. So, what's the best way to do that? We propose that you consider the Mediterranean diet. There are several versions of this diet, but they all emphasize vegetables, fruits, whole grains, legumes, extra-virgin olive oil, nuts, and seeds. Fish and red wine are also included. Numerous studies in recent years have clearly shown that the Mediterranean diet is, at the very least, one of the healthiest diets you can eat.[2]

Finally, A Diet That's Not a Gimmick

Let us count the ways we love the Mediterranean diet:

- It's an incredibly healthy way to eat, now and forever.
- By including so many varied and wonderful foods, it's a sustainable way to eat, now and forever.
- It includes red wine![3]

The Mediterranean diet is highly effective for weight loss,[4] even though it includes a considerable amount of healthy fat, particularly extra-virgin olive oil and nuts. Studies show that eating a Mediterranean diet does not result in weight gain *even if you don't restrict calories.*[5] More than that, though, it's a diet that is sustainable and that has varied health benefits, many of which are due to its effect on your good friend, the intestinal microbiome,[6] protecting you against the chronic inflammation[7, 8] associated with obesity, diabetes, heart disease, arthritis,[9] and impaired brain function.

You can't control your genetic inheritance; you may have inherited genes that increase your risk of getting certain diseases. But you can definitely lower that risk, depending on the way you live. When it comes to weight and disease susceptibility, "although genetic factors play a large role, heritability is not destiny."[10] By changing the foods you eat regularly, you can absolutely change what your future health looks like. This is what the Mediterranean diet has to offer:

1. Weight Loss

In a two-year study comparing the Mediterranean, low-carbohydrate, and low-fat diets, the low-fat group lost the least amount of weight. The Mediterranean diet and low-carbohydrate diets were comparable with regard to weight loss. However, the Mediterranean diet group lost more abdominal fat and had better blood levels of glucose, insulin, and lipids.[11]

2. Metabolic Syndrome Reversal and Type 2 Diabetes Prevention

Metabolic syndrome is a combination of related risk factors for heart disease and type 2 diabetes: high blood pressure, high cholesterol, high triglycerides, high fasting glucose, and abdominal obesity. More than a third of all Americans have metabolic syndrome.[12] If you eat a consistent Mediterranean diet, and especially if you're also physically active, you have the capacity to actually *reverse* all those risk factors.[13]

Type 2 diabetes is often preventable through health benefits and weight loss associated with the Mediterranean diet. Even for people who already have type 2 diabetes, their disease is better controlled if they eat in this way.[14]

3. Heart Disease and Stroke Prevention

Numerous studies have demonstrated the effectiveness of the Mediterranean diet in decreasing the risk of heart disease and stroke.[15, 16, 17] Interestingly, a recent study of people at high risk for cardiovascular disease showed a *protective* benefit on the heart for those who ate a Mediterranean diet with added nuts and extra-virgin olive oil compared to those people who ate a low-fat diet.[18]

Janice—Many of my patients have trouble taking diabetes and hypertension seriously. After all, they're common, painless (at least at first), and invisible. It can be difficult to fully appreciate that these conditions represent a direct line to heart attack and stroke. Heart attack and stroke can sound so far away, and we all have to die of something, right? Well, the big problem may not be dying: with severe heart disease, it's possible to end up being a "cardiac cripple," with the high point of your day being a walk from the bed to the toilet. And life after a stroke? Well, I don't need to tell you what that can look like.

Here's the good news: by losing weight and keeping it off in a healthy way, you will decrease your risk for coronary heart disease by as much as 50 percent and decrease your risk of stroke by 75 percent.[19]

4. Cancer Prevention

Because of the decreased chronic inflammation, the improvement in the body's hormonal balance, and the weight loss itself, staying on a Mediterranean diet lowers your risk of developing cancer, including breast cancer[20] and colon cancer.[21]

5. Improved Brain Health and Prevention of Cognitive Decline

The Mediterranean diet is associated with reduced rates of depression,[22] cognitive decline,[23] and even Alzheimer's Disease.[24] The prevention of cognitive decline and brain atrophy seems particularly related to an increased fish intake and decreased meat intake,[25] as well as an increase in healthy fats, especially extra-virgin olive oil and nuts.[26]

6. Happier Bone and Joints

Extra weight burdens joints and makes it more difficult for you to be physically active. Not surprisingly, weight loss is also associated with a slower progression of osteoarthritis in the knee,[27] as well as a great reduction in lower back pain[28] and other musculoskeletal disorders.[29]

Jae—*When I am analyzing human remains from archaeological sites in the laboratory, I see the effect of heavy, load-bearing labor throughout the skeleton. In my professional setting, I know this is likely due to carrying heavy loads and individuals being subject to culturally specific labor activities in the past (for example, construction, ceramic production, textiles and weaving, food procurement). These same types of changes in the skeleton are seen in modern skeletons too—due to weight bearing from their own body fat.*

To summarize, by eating the right foods, you can decrease your risk of *dying* from the consequences of type 2 diabetes, heart disease, and stroke. The most dramatic decrease is possible if you eat lots of vegetables, fruits, seafood, and nuts and seeds, as well as very little processed meats, sugar-sweetened drinks, and salt. In other words, adhere to the Mediterranean diet, and live a longer, more vital life. Incredibly, even if people don't start the Mediterranean diet until they're over the age of seventy, they still have a 50 percent decrease in mortality over a ten-year period.[30] It's never too late to start! The two of us have largely adopted a Mediterranean diet ourselves, and we urge you to consider it as a change that will bring long-lasting physical and mental health benefits.

Perhaps you want to incorporate the Mediterranean diet into your life gradually—that's fine. Perhaps one meatless dinner a week? One fewer restaurant meal a week? A glass of red wine instead of a shot of vodka? If you're not ready to give up the ice cream yet, that's okay: eat an apple and a few almonds first. See how you feel. Maybe you won't want so much ice cream after that. See what works for you, and be open to making changes. The important thing is for you to feel like you're *adding* something worthwhile to your life that deserves your attention, rather than feeling like you're *giving up* tantalizing, but potentially destructive, foods. This change will become so much easier as you go along with it—we guarantee it.

How Quickly Can Your Body Tolerate Major Changes in Your Diet?

When people go on extreme, restrictive diets, such as very-low-carbohydrate or very-low-calorie diets, they often suffer from headaches, mood changes, hunger, or diarrhea. However, these symptoms should *not* occur when you change from an unhealthy diet to a healthy one. The one caveat has to do with fiber. If you dramatically increase your fiber intake quickly, you may experience bloating and constipation. We recommend that you drink plenty of water and increase the amount of fiber you eat gradually. Give the new healthy bacteria in your intestine time to establish themselves before you consider having lentil stew for lunch and chili for dinner on the same day!

Is It Too Expensive to Eat This Way?

High-quality, fresh, non-processed foods cost more. Grass-fed meat and dairy cost more. Wild salmon costs more. We dispute none of this. But consider other factors, too:

- You don't have to eat wild salmon or grass-fed steak every night. Beans, eggs, soy products, and lentils are all protein-packed. Dinner doesn't have to be a slab of meat with a few vegetables and a potato on the side. In fact, dinner shouldn't look like that at all; rather, it should be a really large portion of colorful vegetables along with some protein and some complex, unrefined carbohydrate such as brown rice or quinoa. A small amount of meat or fish can go a long way when you're eating a mostly plant-based diet. Vegetarian chili is cheap to make, perfect for feeding many people, and easy to freeze (recipe on page 283).

- Restaurant meals, which are less likely to be healthy, are also expensive. Even "moderately" priced restaurants typically end up costing more than a high-quality home-cooked meal.
- Eating unhealthy foods on a regular basis means you're very likely to end up with more medications and more doctor visits. That costs time and money—and not in the way you'd like to spend time and money.

In Chapter 5, we recommended getting store-bought vegetables and fruits that are already cut up if that's what it takes for you to eat produce. Even though it's more expensive, it's a lot better than omitting produce from your diet because you find all that chopping too time-consuming. These are the foods that will keep you healthy, happy, and full. Once again, we want to stress that nutritional supplements, in general, are not a substitute for the wonderful vitamins and minerals that are already in fruits and vegetables. You can pay now or pay later: buy lots of produce in whatever non-processed form you'll eat, and reap the benefits of physical and mental energy—or buy less healthy food for less money now, and spend your money on treating diabetes and heart disease later. And feel crappy.

Jae—I try to remember that everything I am doing has a long-term effect. I'm investing not only in my present self, but also in my future. I'd rather spend more money on healthy food and less money on eating out so often. It feels good to take my future into my own hands.

Here are a few examples of delicious, fiber-rich, inexpensive meals you can consider:

Breakfast: oatmeal with berries and chopped nuts
Lunch: black bean burger; salad with tomatoes, cucumbers, and white beans
Dinner: lentil soup, chili, or whole-grain pasta with spinach, mushrooms, and zucchini

It's hard to give up processed, manufactured foods. They're convenient, delicious, and ubiquitous. You might remember our quote in Chapter 4 from the book *The Evolution of Obesity:* "We evolved on the savannahs of Africa; we now live in Candyland."[31] It's now time to evolve some more.

STEP FOUR:

Make Success Inevitable

CHAPTER 9

Transforming Your Kitchen from a Danger Zone into a Safe Space

---

Merely seeing or smelling a desired food may make you "hungrier" for that food, even if you're not actually hungry.

Have these scenarios ever happened to you?

- You come home at the end of the day, tired and ravenous. You open the refrigerator and start stabbing at the leftover Chinese food. You open the cupboard to see if there are any chips left. Cook dinner? You're too frazzled to even think about that.
- There's a cookie jar on the counter labeled "For the kids." Sure.
- You open the freezer to take out frozen fruit, but the ice cream is staring at you.
- There's nothing in the house for dinner, so you just order in pizza. Again.

These examples represent traps that will likely derail your best efforts to change the way you eat. It's time for a kitchen make-over. No, we're not talking about granite countertops—we're talking about what's *on* your countertop. Is there a bowl of fruit or a cookie jar? What's in the cupboard—a bag of nuts or a bag of chips? A can of beans or a can of creamed corn? A box of oatmeal or a box of choco-marshmallow crispies?

How about the refrigerator? Is there a supply of apples and carrots or bottles of soda and half a pie? And your freezer? Do you see frozen soup in ready-to-serve portions or a smorgasbord of ice cream containers?

If your go-to foods in the kitchen are mostly convenience food in boxes, it's time to make that space work *for* you and not *against* you. Make a plan, develop a strategy for sharing that plan with other household members, and carry it out.

Not surprisingly, the kitchen is the most important room in your house for everything we've been talking about in this book. It's not just the room where you store, prepare, and eat food—it's also where the triggers are, and it's where you'll take control of your future. We want to give you tools for success so you can transform your kitchen from a battle zone to a safe haven.

Are We All Just a Bunch of Pavlov's Dogs?

The brain reacts to the sight and smell of tasty food. For example, when you smell something delicious, you may salivate. That's a normal, physiologic response—it's not learned behavior.[1] But things are not as simple as just that. In the nineteenth century, Ivan Pavlov performed an experiment where he rang a bell at the same time he put food out for the dogs; in response, they salivated. Eventually, merely ringing the bell induced salivation, even if he didn't give the dogs food (poor dogs). This is called a *conditioned response*, and humans have conditioned responses, too. Merely seeing or smelling a desired food may make you "hungrier" for that food, even if you're not actually hungry.[2] It's a learned, conditioned response that is associated with weight gain.[3]

Trigger Foods: Tantalizing Traps

Trigger foods undermine your best-laid plans to eat in a calm, intentional way. They are associated with those conditioned responses, or food cues, that inevitably lead to cravings (to which we've devoted nearly all of Chapter 14) and uncontrolled eating. No matter how much you try to practice self-control, any hope of eating these foods "in moderation" may be simply out of the question for you.

For the two of us, our triggers are sugary and/or fatty processed foods like cookies, chips, and ice cream. What are yours? And what do you do with them? Ideally, these diabolical temptations shouldn't be in your house. You're just asking for trouble, and why do that to yourself? But if you're not ready to banish the chips—it may seem like too much to ask of yourself, at least for now, and we get that—then we suggest that whenever you find yourself wanting a bowl of chips, at least have an apple first. Fill up your stomach with something healthy, and give yourself time to feel less desperate about the chips. Better yet, walk out of the kitchen, and see if you can distract yourself with something that isn't food.

Janice—If there's a cookie jar on the counter and I'm hungry or "just in the mood," what do you think is going to happen? Telling myself "just say no" or "I'll have just one" is ludicrous and impossible. It's also unfair to me to set myself up for that kind of frustration and failure. If, instead, there's a bowl of apples on the counter, I'll reach for an apple if I'm actually hungry and be done with it. No cue. No trigger. No craving. No loss of control. No disappointment in myself.

Jae—*If you recall my "lowest point," which I wrote about in the introduction, you'll remember my night of pizza, breadsticks, and ice cream. Wanting to eat like that was, and still is, my fundamental problem: I do not fully understand hunger cues, even after my 140-pound weight loss. There is a large disconnect between my brain and my stomach. They are not in sync with each other, which makes this whole "healthy eating" thing tough. Some people can eat half a plate of food, then push it away and declare, "I'm full; I don't want any more." I am so jealous of that. Being able to leave delicious food on a plate feels like a superpower I wish I had.*

Even if I promise to keep a trigger food, say chips, all the way in the back of the pantry, wrapped in two bags and hiding in an old oatmeal container, there always comes a time that my Evil Twin cons me into thinking I can have "just one." Right.

While eliminating trigger foods from your house may be ideal, if you don't feel ready to rid your kitchen of all the unhealthy foods you still love, put them in a much less accessible cupboard or down in the basement. At least you'll have to make an effort to reach them. Our personal system of all or nothing may not be necessary for you at all. There's not just one way, and it can take some time to figure out what will work best for you. Open your cupboards and consider which foods would be really hard to throw out and why. But if it's something like a six-pack box of chips, five of which you ate yesterday, then maybe that's a trigger food and you're better off just not letting them into your home.

What if the kitchen is not completely your domain? What if other household members are unwilling to part with their chips? This is the time to have a discussion. Be direct with them, but be open to listen to their side, too. Are they willing to keep the chips away from your sight? Can they eat chips only when they're out of the house (for example, keeping a bag at the office instead of your shared pantry)? Explain that this is really important to you and that you *expect* their support. There should be no negative comments, no teasing, and no undermining. See what you can negotiate—have a discussion, advocate strongly for your position, and be willing to listen to their points of view.

Now check out your refrigerator. Wouldn't it be nice if there were some carrot and celery sticks or red pepper slices ready for you and your family or housemates to grab when they want a little snack? Wouldn't it be nice to keep fruit that keeps for a while, like apples and oranges, in the produce drawer? Turn the healthy foods into *convenience* foods that everyone will reach for first. Perhaps it will work for you to keep the less healthy foods in the back of the refrigerator where they won't have so loud a voice when you're looking for a quick snack.

Janice—I always keep fruit in the refrigerator or out on the counter. I make sure there are carrot sticks or steamed string beans ready for munching while I cook dinner. There's usually a pot of soup or a batch of roasted vegetables that I made over the weekend and can polish off during the week. You get the picture. If I come home from work and I'm tired and cranky, and the only choice I have is either to chop, measure, and cook or just open a cupboard and grab a box of something crunchy and salty and sweet, guess what's more likely to happen? That's why healthy food has to be ready for me. I'm like almost everyone else—I want to have food that is readily available and convenient, which is why it's no wonder that prepackaged processed foods are so abundant. But depending on those foods is not the way that I want to care for myself. I am committed to having a fitter, slimmer, healthier body. I deserve that.

Jae—*Me, too. When I cook all my meals ahead of time on Sundays, there's little last-minute prep involved, and I'm more likely to eat something healthy throughout the week.*

The same idea applies to your cupboards and pantry. Make your space work *for* you. Stock up on spices and seasonings so that you can make vegetables taste more interesting and flavorful. Fill up the space with dried or canned beans, whole grains, lentils, and oatmeal. Keep some nuts, seeds, and dried fruit for snacks. Herbal teas often have a slightly sweet taste and are very soothing. As you try new foods and recipes, you'll recognize what ingredients you want to keep on hand.

Whether you work inside or outside the home, or you're a student studying crazy hours or a stay-at-home parent, the freezer is your best friend because it allows you to store food that you've cooked ahead for a long time. Consider, for example, making a large supply of soup or chili or stew whenever you have some free time, and then freeze the food in smaller-size portion containers. Prepare yourself for success!

Kids in the Kitchen

If you're a parent or you live with other family members, invite your family into the kitchen to prepare food and cook together. Kids love to eat what they have helped to cook. If you're lucky, this might even apply to teenagers. How much nicer to spend a rainy Sunday afternoon cooking with them than having them sit in front of a screen without talking at all?

Step Away from Danger

Here's a strategy to consider when you're *not* preparing food or eating a meal: get the heck out of the kitchen. Do something else, and think about something else. Literally walk away from that place in your home where you think you *have* to have a bowl of ice cream right this second and that nothing else matters.

Jae—*For me, the kitchen is a place that gives me a lot of anxiety. This isn't surprising, since it's where all the food is, and it holds something that I have historically had difficulty with. I know this and I'm aware of it, so I make sure that whenever I have to go through my kitchen for something other than for prepping or eating a meal, I walk through without stopping. This helps me avoid mindless eating when I'm not physically hungry. After I prepare food, I try to leave the kitchen to actually eat the food. I leave the serving dish in the kitchen and take my plate into another room in order to eat. This way, it's less convenient to get a second helping—and I also have time to think about whether I really want it.*

In fact, I go an extra step further. After I serve myself, I put all the food back in their respective containers and in the fridge. For example, one of my favorite dishes to make for myself is vegetable stir-fry. Whenever I prepare veggie stir-fry, I usually make a lot because I can always reheat the leftovers for other meals. Then, instead of leaving the food in the pan or in one big container, I portion it out right away into meal sizes so that they're all ready to go for future meals. Then I take the plate I served myself and go into the other room to eat. Since the stir-fry is already put away, I'm not able to continuously and mindlessly serve myself more food; I know I'll have to make an extra effort to go back to the kitchen, take the food out, reheat it, and then return to the table. If I'm legitimately hungry, then there's nothing wrong with getting more food. However, if I'm just eating for some sort of instant gratification, the best way to stop that bad habit is to create all those extra steps that

97

make getting that second helping not worth it. Additionally, the extra steps buy me time—time to reconsider if this is what I actually want and if I'm actually hungry. It gives me time to make the healthier, more loving choice for myself and my body.

This extends to things like chips and candy and ice cream—since I do not have them in my house, I'll have to physically leave and go somewhere else to purchase them. I've promised myself that if I do want a cookie or an ice cream, I'll have to walk to the store that's about two miles away to get it. That gives me about forty minutes to really think through what I'm about to do, and make sure that I am making a rational decision. If I get to the store and still want the ice cream, then at least I've walked four miles round-trip to think about my options. If I don't want to walk that far, then I really don't need the ice cream in the first place.

Janice—No wonder Jae remains such an inspiration to me!

CHAPTER 10

Success Is Not an Accident

Does it take me a while to make my lunch?
Yes, about fifteen minutes longer. . . . Do
I want the few minutes of sleep more than
I want to do what it takes to feel
great about myself? No way.

Consider these scenarios:

- It's 10:30 a.m., and it's already been a tough morning at work. You go into the break room to make a cup of tea, and you see an open box of donuts. You're in a bad mood, and your lunch hour isn't for another hour and a half, so what the heck? After lunch, since you've already blown your diet, you stop by the desk of a coworker who's a total pain but who always has a jar of candy on her desk.
- You go out to lunch with your friends and order the same thing they do—a cheeseburger with fries and a soda.
- You go to a meeting—a meeting in which you have no interest whatsoever—but you go anyway because you know there will be free pizza.

In the examples we listed above, the choices regarding food were impulsive and random. **Planning ahead**, on the other hand, is a strategy that allows you to eat foods you have rationally chosen with a sense of calm pleasure and respect for your body. We cannot overstate its value in our continued success.

Planning Instead of Wishing

Planning prevents you from ambushing yourself when some external situation threatens to undermine your intentions. Planning helps you enjoy food in a manner that is intentional and deliberate. You no longer need to quickly wolf down food in a secretive, guilt-ridden, emotionally desperate way. You no longer need to tell yourself, "I'll try not to eat more than that," only to realize ten minutes later that you've eaten *way* more than that. We want to offer you a way to plan what you're going to eat ahead of time and then carry out that plan. Enjoy the food, congratulate yourself for sticking to your intention and for taking care of yourself, and then move on, preferably to non-food-related activities. This strategy represents a major paradigm shift: moving from emotional, impulsive eating to a rational, tranquil enjoyment of food.

Janice—*I've now worked with hundreds of patients regarding food issues, and they have all identified planning as a key element for helping them to lose weight and sustain the weight loss. As for myself, now that I've learned to plan ahead, I find that I've eliminated all the stress and anxiety that was associated with eating. There's no longer that exhausting inner dialogue that used to play out with every meal or snack. I'm sure you know what I mean: "I know that I shouldn't have a third helping of lasagna, but maybe just this once," or, "I'm really full, but that cake looks so good." Instead, I now decide ahead* of time what I'm going to eat and how much, and then I enjoy every single bite.

Jae—It's hard to express how much meal planning has changed my life, not only while I was in the process of losing weight, but also in the four years that I have maintained my weight. Planning what I'm going to eat ahead of time lets me eat in a sane, calm way, especially when it comes to portion control.

Practicing self-care did not stop when I fit into that one size or hit that one number. This kind of thoughtfulness is something I'll probably need to (and want to) work on forever. Meal preparation is a tool that lets me work on my relationship with food, and I plan to keep up the practice. I can envision myself preparing my lunches ahead of time throughout grad school, when I have a family, and even when I'm retired—I know it's something I can keep as part of my daily life to help me maintain a healthy relationship with my food and with my body.

Meal Prep: An Assembly Line of Self-Care

For both of us, preparing meals or parts of meals ahead of time is an essential component of our continued healthy weight-loss success. If we don't bring lunch with us to work or school, we may be tempted to grab a burger and fries. When we come home at the end of a long day, washing and chopping vegetables may sound like a time-consuming, optional task. So, here's how we deal with food prep in a way that works for us.

Breakfast

Breakfast is an important meal for most people, as we'll discuss in Chapter 22. However, neither of us eat breakfast, other than perhaps a spoonful of yogurt. This is not a strategy we necessarily recommend; it's just what works for us. Here's a strategy that doesn't work for anyone, though: giving yourself ten minutes to get out the door and just throwing a breakfast pastry in the toaster while you put on your shoes. Please don't do that.

Instead, if you don't have time to sit down for breakfast, consider taking with you a hard-boiled egg that you've prepared ahead of time. Or take a minute to make a smoothie (check out our recipe on page 305) or whip one up the night before. Or take a few minutes to eat some yogurt or oatmeal (you can even make overnight oatmeal) with berries and nuts.

Lunch

Jae—First, I want to share how meal prep helps me and explain why it's worth the time it takes. Then, I'll walk you through one of my typical weeks to give you a better idea of how this plays out in real life. Finally, you can decide for yourself if you want to incorporate this system into your life.

Here's what my meal preparation looks like: I do my planning, shopping, and cooking on Sundays. I like to devote Saturdays to friends and doing fun things, and then reserve Sunday as a day to start getting into the mindset of preparing for the week to come. I eat the same thing for lunch almost every day, and that works for me.

For example, one Sunday I was feeling tuna and decided to incorporate that into my lunches for the week. I chose a tuna salad recipe that could easily be prepared in one big batch and then divided it into smaller portions. I then wrote a list of all the ingredients I needed and went to the store, taking care to stick to my predetermined list. When I got home, I mashed up three avocados, chopped up an onion, diced two tomatoes, and squeezed in lime. I mixed all of this with five cans of tuna, divided the mixture into five containers, topped it with sriracha sauce, and then put the containers in the fridge.

As you can see, my lunches were packed with protein from the tuna, contained vegetables, and had creamy deliciousness and healthy fat from the avocado. I also packed three whole grain crackers to add something crunchy and interesting to my tuna salad. Finally, I packed an apple so I could have something sweet to finish off the meal. In all, at the end of the one hour it took me to prep my food, I had five lunches ready to go for the week.

Janice—*Gee, Jae, our lunches are awfully similar! I do mine a little differently. I bring the same lunch every day to work, but I usually make lunch each morning. I'm a morning person—I love to get up really, really early (and go to bed really, really early; you'd think I was a farmer), and so making lunch at that time of day is easy for me. And, believe it or not, it's kind of relaxing. It's a nice way to start the day knowing that I'm taking good care of myself.*

The part I do ahead is to make a vinaigrette that's two-thirds extra-virgin olive oil and one-third balsamic vinegar. If I'm feeling wild and crazy, I might add a little mustard. I make enough to last for a week or so and keep it in a jar in the refrigerator.

I put a lot of greens (spinach and/or arugula and/or kale, plus some romaine lettuce) into a big plastic container. I add a protein, such as a can of tuna or salmon, or fish or chicken from the night before. Sometimes, I go vegetarian and use chickpeas or black beans. I rinse and drain canned beans because they're so convenient. Next, it's time for some chopped-up carrots and/or jicama, maybe some steamed string beans or asparagus, and avocado. I might add chopped walnuts or pumpkin seeds, too. I toss everything with a little of the vinaigrette that I've made. Finally, I pack little bags of almonds, carrots, and apple or pear slices so I have snacks when I need them.

Does it take me a while to make my lunch? Yes, about fifteen minutes. Do I sometimes wish I could sleep fifteen minutes longer in the morning? Yes. Do I want the few minutes of sleep more than I want to do what it takes to feel great about myself? No way.

Jae—I will admit that food planning and preparation are time-consuming. I need to make a list, shop, prep, cook, and store my food. In my case, this is usually to make a week's worth of food. Like everyone else, I have a busy life. At first, I wondered if it was worth it, or even possible, to set aside the time to do all that. But believe me, when I get an extra fifteen minutes of sleep in the morning because my lunches are already packed, and when I come home from work and most of my dinner is ready to just heat up, I'm so relieved that I took the time on the weekend to do the work beforehand.

Perhaps you don't share our intense love of salads. No problem. Make a big batch of a one-pot meal and reheat portions for lunch. And if you don't want to prepare your lunches, see if you can find a healthy, delicious lunch place near your work where you can eat in or take out. There are some truly amazing soup and salad bar places in most towns and cities.

Dinner

Jae—I don't necessarily meal prep or cook at home every dinner because life happens and there are nights when I work late or something unexpected comes up. In order not to waste money, when I do cook dinners in advance, I usually prepare two or three dinners at once. Even though many of my dinners are relatively unplanned, I still make sure that my food purchases are conducive to healthy eating habits so I won't sabotage myself when I need to "improvise" my meal. My system allows for variety in my food and helps me feel like I'm not restricting myself. I still have to be—and want *to be—mindful of each of my food choices, but this bit of freedom is what I need in order to help me stick with my overall plan.*

Janice—*For me, the most important part of dinner is making sure that I'm going to have lots of vegetables on hand. I usually roast a big batch of vegetables early in the week and eat them for several days, either on their own or mixed with grains. Or I make a big pot of vegetable soup. Or I have microwavable string beans in a bag. You see what I mean. The vegetables are the anchor for whatever else I eat.*

Jae—*I love soup, too. It's 1) easy to make, 2) easy to split up into serving sizes, 3) easy to freeze, and 4) easy to heat up. I usually spend two hours on a Sunday making a huge batch that I freeze into twenty portions. That means I have twenty "safety nets." If I find myself in a bind where I didn't plan ahead, I don't even have to worry about whether or not I'll be pressured into making the right choice because, guess what? I just open the freezer, heat up my healthy soup, and congratulate myself because I had planned ahead, followed through, and set myself up for success.*

A pro tip for freezing soups: freeze them in muffin tins. Once the soup is solid, you can take out the individual portions and put them into a freezer bag. This allows you to easily defrost as many "soup muffins" as you want at a time.

I also love to freeze egg-based dishes. A really simple thing I prepare in individual servings is my "egg bake." After I bake it, I cut it into slices that are the right size for a sandwich and put each piece in a sandwich bag, which then goes into a freezer bag right into the freezer. Then, whenever I like, I take out a slice, pop it in the microwave, and have an instant egg and vegetable sandwich.

Gather the Children!

Janice—I'd like to say something about shopping, prepping, and cooking on weekends for people with children. Maybe there's laundry, studying, kids' soccer games, church, a night out. Food shopping, prepping, and cooking may seem like a lot to add to the mix. I would suggest that if you have children, consider doing much of this with them. Let them help you choose the most gorgeous apples or berries. Teach them to decipher food labels. When you get home, let them help with meal prep. You can set them a contest to make a meal that has the most colors (gummy bears don't count!). If they're young, get them a plastic kids' knife and let them cut off strawberry tops. Older kids who help to cook learn fractions when they measure ingredients, as well as other kitchen skills—and most of all, they'll be spending time with you. This is time they won't be staring at a screen of one sort or another; instead, this family time together with result in several healthy meals packed away in the refrigerator or freezer. What's more, kids tend to love eating the food that they've prepared. You don't have to tell them how healthy it is!

We hope you can easily apply our ideas and experiences at home. Going out to eat, though, is much tougher. In a restaurant, for example, you may experience all sorts of "food cues"—conditioned responses that make you intensely desire certain foods when they're right in front of you, such as warm bread. We'll get to eating out in detail in Chapter 20. For now, suffice to say that planning ahead is really, really going to help you when it comes to eating out. If you're going out to lunch with your coworkers, for example, try to make sure you're dining at a place with food that's both healthy and satisfying for you by going online and checking the menu before you leave your office. Think about, and decide ahead of time, if you're going to have a piece of bread or some dessert at the restaurant. By taking the time to consciously plan ahead and commit to that plan, you can enjoy every sip and every bite that passes through your lips.

Don't Give Your Evil Twin a Place at the Table

You can see the importance we place on planning and structure. Spontaneity is not your friend in the process of changing your relationship with food and your body. But does planning what you're going to eat ahead of time prevent you from experiencing the joy of eating? Absolutely not! In fact, it's just the opposite—planning affords you the opportunity to savor your food without the Evil Twin having a seat at the table. Having said that, structure is not meant to be rigid or punitive. For example, be sure to schedule in time for people and activities that you enjoy. Those aren't luxuries!

Janice—*I've got to tell you, I sometimes have a lot of anxiety, but planning ahead is the reason I don't have anxiety around food anymore. And to me, that is simply incredible.*

CHAPTER 11

Putting Your Action Plan to Work

> Setbacks are an inevitable part of the
> process of weight loss, but caustic
> self-criticism does not have to be.

We hope you've identified your personal motivators for committing to healthy eating by now. You've outlined goals that are *your* goals, and you've considered ways to effectively shut down the negative, discouraging "Evil Twin" voice in your head. Now it's time to put your personalized goals into action.

Use Short-Term Goals to Get Long-Term Results

Back in Chapter 3, we talked about the importance of setting goals for yourself. Goals should be positive, specific, measurable, and, most of all, *achievable*. When your goals are defined in this way, not only do you increase your prospects for success, but your achievements also build on one another to create a new reality. A study of overweight men and women showed that "setting small, achievable behavior change goals" led to greater weight loss.[1] It's all a matter of maximizing opportunities for success and making those successes cumulative.

Jae—*As I talked about in Chapter 1, once I finally made the commitment to change my lifestyle and habits, I seriously examined my "ultimate goal" of losing a hundred pounds. That goal did not help me at all with figuring out where to begin. The idea of losing a hundred pounds was so overwhelming—it's an incredibly large number! It was apparent to me that I had to reevaluate how to make my goal more achievable and realistic. That was how I decided to think about losing a hundred pounds as losing one pound a week—and doing it a hundred times. Essentially, I identified my ultimate goal and found a way to chip it down into smaller, manageable pieces—I knew I could figure out what to do to lose just one pound per week, and I knew it was something realistic I could achieve that would give me the satisfaction of accomplishing what I'd set out to do in regular intervals. Reframing my goal in this way ensured that I would not feel so frustrated and overwhelmed by the number 100. In doing this, I created a very powerful tool that allowed me to turn my aspirations into a reality.*

I remember the night clearly. I was an eighteen-year-old college freshman. I sat at my desk in my college dorm room. I was introverted and lonely, and I weighed 270 pounds. I opened my bright-pink planner and wrote the number "1" on the top-left corner of the page next to Monday, January 14, 2013. I turned the page to display a new week and wrote a "2" next to January 21—another page-turn and I wrote "3" next to January 28. This process repeated until I reached "100" next to Monday, December 15, 2014. I underlined the "100" and drew a large square around it, put down the pen, and leaned back in my chair with my arms folded. I had created my roadmap.

Janice—*I love how Jae worked out her strategy. It's the best response to what a patient of mine once said to me: "The long-term goals feel so far away, and the short-term goals don't seem worth it." In fact, though, short-term goals really are essential to prevent you from experiencing what my college-age patients refer to as "rage quit," when they quit in a state of rage toward the person or book or commercial that recommended yet another unsustainable or even ludicrous diet. And then you feel rage toward yourself. On the other hand, reaching short-term goals and building from one to the next is, in fact, precisely what will ultimately get you to the long-term prize.*

For me personally, I have a long-term goal of eating in an intentional, healthy way. Clearly, that's a lot easier said than done. If there are cookies in my house, then I am going to eat all the cookies. Period. I know this. So in order to achieve my long-term goal, there can simply be no cookies in the house. How can I make that happen? I have found that what works for me is to break down that long-term goal into several smaller, short-term ones. For example, before I even walk into the supermarket, I tell myself that my goal is simply to skip the cookie aisle. Then, once I'm in the store, I actually walk right past that Aisle of False Promises. Success!

__Jae__—Remember that this is not a diet! If you want to make a change for the rest of your life, it's important to keep in mind that this is about change in how you think and how you live.

The small changes I made while I was losing weight did not always seem linear and purposeful in the moment. But after I lost all the weight, I could see that the aggregation of small changes added up to a 142-pound loss. I thought to myself, I can't imagine living my life like I used to, and I'm not going to.

Figure Out Your Short-Term Goals

In order to maximize your opportunities for success, make sure that when you think about these short-term goals, you do so when you're in a positive mindset. There is evidence that people who write about their goals with optimism are less likely to become self-critical.[2]

List #5: Short-Term Goals

If you're having a hard time thinking of ways to break down your ultimate goal into smaller chunks, here are some examples of short-term goals that we've set for ourselves. You may want to refer to these for inspiration.

Janice's list
- *Today, I will try to catch myself when I notice a self-critical thought and will reframe that thought into something positive.*
- *Today, every time I make a decision regarding healthy food or physical activity, I will congratulate myself for a job well done.*
- *I will exercise when I get home from work today.*
- *I will not eat anything after dinner tonight, unless it's a vegetable or a fruit.*
- *I will eat no refined sugar today.*
- *I will walk for half an hour today before I make dinner.*

Jae's list
- *I'm going to hit my "move" goal on my Apple Watch today.*
- *When I make healthy food choices this weekend, I will not "congratulate" myself by eating something that is unhealthy.*
- *I will not sit in bed and watch Netflix as soon as I get in the door after work this week.*
- *I'm going to the gym tonight, even if I'm a little tired.*
- *I will brush my teeth at 8.00 p.m. tonight to help me stop night snacking.*
- *I am going to remove all the snacks from my car.*

Set Yourself Up for Success

It's up to you to decide what a "short-term" goal means. Some days will be a lot harder than others. If you find yourself in one of those days, your short-term goals might be just to get through dining at this one restaurant without ordering French fries or going on this one grocery store trip without putting ice cream into the cart. Then, thank yourself and celebrate the victory. Because it truly is a victory.

Maybe your short-term goal is to skip the second cocktail tonight or to take the stairs up a flight or two instead of the elevator. Eventually, you may want the goals to be more substantive, such as committing to a goal of taking three brisk walks one week; or making yourself healthy lunches for the next work week; or brushing your teeth immediately after dinner every night; or eliminating soda from your house. You decide—they're your goals to define, and you are the one who has to stick with them. Just be sure that the goals, in addition to being meaningful for you, are achievable. How great will it be when you are successful? If the overarching goal is to eat and move in a physically and emotionally healthy way, then you can start to incorporate that goal into your daily routine right now—you can already be *living* your goal.

Jae—The roadmap I made for myself of losing a single pound a hundred times was an approach that allowed me to stay on track and hold myself accountable in the two years that followed, starting from that night with the planner. My approach worked for me, played to my personal strengths, and worked with my lifestyle. I hope that seeing my process, and how small the initial short-term goals were and how effective the result was, will give you hope. It's okay to not know where to start, and it's okay to set a goal just for this day, this hour, or this minute—the important thing is that you have made a commitment to change your relationship with your body, and that's a commitment worth celebrating.

Give Yourself Credit

Imagine this: you go for a walk after work instead of just turning on the television. This happened because you made a choice—you set a goal, and you achieved the goal. You know you can do it again. Pause for a moment, and congratulate yourself. Thank yourself for taking care of yourself and for carrying out your intentions. Think about how your body is thanking you. This is success.

No matter how small the goal you set or how small the change you make, be sure to acknowledge each one and give yourself a pat on the back. For example:

- You make oatmeal for breakfast instead of grabbing a croissant at the local coffee shop.
- You stop at the gym on your way home from work.
- You go to the grocery store, skip the snack aisle, and stock up on fruit.
- You make a walking date instead of a lunch date with a friend.
- You have one glass of wine with dinner instead of two.

None of these activities is earth-shattering or life-changing in itself, but each is worthy of pausing to celebrate a job well done. No, we're not being ridiculous, and we're not telling you to congratulate yourself for simply breathing, either. But we *are* saying that shifting away from a deprivation mindset to one in which you feel accomplished and optimistic will make all the difference in the world to your being able to stay on your path to good habits, good health, and well-being. We cannot overstate the value of feeling successful, strong, and proud of yourself and how it contributes to making your successes cumulative and permanent.

We recommend that you do even more than say "good job" to yourself. Write down every victory, including the small ones. Sure, going down a pants size is a success, but so is eating fish instead of ribs for dinner. Here is your next list.

List #6: Your Victories

The reason that every success, no matter how small, is worth acknowledging and celebrating is that it's the *process* of achieving success and getting closer to your ultimate goal that counts. Ultimately, it's taking care of yourself that counts.

Janice—*I love how one of my patients put it to me: "I look at My Fitness Pal at the end of each day and see how I did. And then I say, 'Good job, Charlotte.' That means that every day, I'm proud of myself."*

Reward Yourself When You Reach a Goal

We've emphasized that a feeling of deprivation is guaranteed to sabotage your efforts to change how you eat. There simply must be continuous rewards along the way, in addition to the obvious one of weight loss. In fact, weight loss isn't sufficient in itself as a reward—if it were, then 80 percent of the people who lose weight wouldn't gain it back!

Jae—*I've heard many suggestions from people about how they reward themselves when hitting certain benchmarks. Some people buy new workout clothes, which motivates them to go to the gym. I know a girl who had a charm bracelet and who would add another charm whenever she hit a certain milestone. Someone else got a tattoo when she reached her goal weight to symbolize everything she had accomplished. For these people, the visual reinforcement, not food, was motivating as they worked toward their goals.*

***Janice**—For me, the ongoing positive feedback I give myself is a tremendous reward in itself (I think I'll skip the tattoo!). Having said that, I enjoy tangible rewards as well. I reward myself by getting new songs for my exercise playlist or buying special fruits, like Asian pears—even if they're not on sale. Or by getting a new shirt to go with the pants that I can finally zip.*

The point is, frequent rewards are an important part of the process of changing your relationship with food *forever*. Don't wait until there's a large weight loss before you care about how you look and how you present yourself to the world. Reward yourself with new beauty products now. Buy a new business suit that makes you feel confident now—you can always have it altered later. Most important, don't wait for weight loss to end the shame. You have the capacity to end the shame right now. Give yourself permission.

The Opposite of Reward Should Not Be Punishment

What if you don't meet your goal? What if you ate ice cream after dinner though you had set a goal not to? Are you a failure? No, you are not a failure—you ate ice cream, that's all. Perhaps your goal simply wasn't realistic at the time. An "achievable" goal means it's achievable for *you*. Reflect on what happened. What was the barrier? Was it because there was ice cream in the house and you heard it calling to you from inside the freezer? Was it that you thought you could watch everyone in your family eat a sundae after dinner while you had strawberries?

In order for this goal to be truly achievable for you, perhaps the ice cream has to go—at least for now. Maybe your family has to eat ice cream only outside the house. Or—everyone eats strawberries for dessert at home (which is a good thing anyway)! People who have the most success with weight loss are those who focus on actively making good choices and not just avoiding bad ones.[3]

Once you've figured out how your plan got derailed and you've taken steps to respond to that, such as getting rid of the ice cream at home, you're readying yourself for your next achievable goal. There's no place for telling yourself that you're lacking willpower or that you can't do this. Neither is true. Starting right now, you'll have many other opportunities for success. In fact, you've transformed this misstep into cause for celebration: you slipped and then you got back up. Now, rewind the clock to zero.

Promise yourself now that if you have a slipup, you won't respond with ugly thoughts and words that you would never hurl at another human being. If you mess up, please don't tell yourself, "I blew it. I failed today, so I'll just keep eating crap and maybe start again tomorrow." Don't keep yourself in that negative space for the rest of the day. It's not one day at a time—rather, it's one *choice* at a time. What you ate an hour ago has nothing to do with what you're going to eat next. You can make a positive choice about what you're going to eat from this moment forward—and that's another opportunity for success.

Don't let a misstep go to waste—learn from it. Setbacks are an inevitable part of the process of weight loss, but caustic self-criticism does not have to be. In fact, there's evidence that people who face setbacks with *less* judgment are *more* likely to achieve long-lasting weight loss.[4]

STEP FIVE:

Be Your Own Best Advocate

CHAPTER 12

You Don't Need to Do This Alone

Being part of a supportive and committed community was incredibly helpful and beneficial in helping me to stick with my plans.

Using food to soothe emotional pain and shame is a tough process to undo—we don't need to tell you that. In this chapter, we'll help you identify your own specific sources of **strength and support** to assist you in changing your relationship with food. Now for the next list:

Your Strengths

What are you good at? What do other people view as your strengths? What are the "non-strengths" you wish to work on? Here are some of our own answers:

Janice's list:

My two strengths and one "non-strength" have helped me so much in my process of losing weight and keeping it off.

Strength 1: *I value independence highly and work hard to do what it takes to take care of myself.*
Strength 2: *I am a compassionate person as a physician, family member, and friend.*

These strengths came together at my "stepladder moment," when I decided to turn my life around. My physical discomfort made me worried about my future independence. At the same time, it dawned on me that hating myself for being in my predicament would not help me lose weight and that it was time to extend compassion to myself for a change and not only to other people.

And it worked. I'm truly okay with who I am. I'm truly okay with my quite-old body. I'm looking forward to a fit future.

Jae's list:
My two strengths have helped me as well.
Strength 1: *I am a competitive person, but I'm mostly competitive with myself. This has helped me to achieve academic success and to have very high aspirations for myself. I function best when I have a goal to help me stay persistent and motivated. Also, my style of learning is methodical, analytical, and visual. When I was ready to lose weight, I learned everything I could about healthy lifestyle change, I kept data, and I collected pictures. This is how I built success on success and tailored my goals as I gained knowledge about what worked best for me. All my strategies were related to making sustainable life changes. I knew that if I didn't do it this way, I would get frustrated and never achieve my aspirations.*
Strength 2: *I am a visual person. While looking for tattoo ideas on Pinterest, I found the photo of a plus-size woman who was curvy—even thick—and the embodiment of a sexy-looking, well-nourished woman. She was a healthy weight, covered in ink, and wearing only a bra and*

panties as she stood looking out the window—with nothing suggestive or seductive about her pose at all. I remember thinking that she just looked so confident and beautiful. She became my "inspiration"—I wanted to look like her. There was something about how she carried herself that exuded confidence and ownership of her body and that was so incredibly appealing to me.

Now, it's your turn. What are your sources of inner strength that you can use in the process of changing your relationship with food?

List #7: Your Strengths

We'll bet that you have more strengths than you realize. Here's a visual: suppose you are on a flight of stairs that has ten steps, and you're only on the third step. You look up, and it doesn't seem possible that you can get yourself to the top. How do you get from the third step to the fourth? You don't feel strong enough. Now, let's reframe this situation. How did you get from the second step to the third? You were successful at that. You have been in many difficult situations in the past where you used perseverance, intelligence, and courage that you didn't even know you had. Think about them, list them, and draw on them for support.

Your Supports

There are very, very few accomplishments that don't involve the help and support of others. This is not a sign of weakness, but rather an understanding that we all gain strength from interdependence, connection, and support. Your sources of support will strengthen your resolve and continued motivation.

Support from Family or Other Household Members

Your living environment plays a big role in your ability to reach your goals. If you have roommates, they may have food in the house that you don't want around. If you live with your family, you may be dependent on your parents or other relatives when it comes to what foods are in the house and what meals are prepared. If you live with a partner and/or if you have children, you need to address their food preferences and health concerns. We get that, and we can help you with these issues.

If you don't live alone, it is vital to communicate with the other people in your home. You will need to ask for support from your family or other housemates about what food is currently in the house and what food should ideally be in the house in order to support your decision to eat in a better way. Do not worry about coming across as demanding or controlling. You are neither of these things—rather, you are simply advocating for your own well-being. This can be good for them, too! Does your roommate want to have communal chocolate in the house? Then ask him if he would be willing to store it somewhere away from the kitchen—and to keep that location a secret. Or consider this possibility—does he absolutely *have* to have chocolate in the house? Maybe he can go out and get it from the convenience store around the block whenever he wants. Be firm when stating your needs—but don't forget to be calm and open to negotiation while doing so.

Janice—Here's the compromise that I made with my cookie-loving family: Fig Newtons. They're the only cookie I've never liked—but my family thinks they're pretty good. So that's what we keep in the house. A win-win for everyone.

Shaming vs. Support

Make sure to address how much adopting a healthy lifestyle means to you, and how important it is that you get their support throughout the process. If this makes you nervous, sit down and think about (then write out) what their support means in your own context. Reflecting on these things ahead of time can help you think through possible scenarios and how you would like them to ideally play out. Share your thoughts with others, in advance when possible. For example, imagine you waver and eat a piece of cake, and your mom "catches" you. Suppose she says, "I thought you said you weren't going to eat cake." You need to recognize that this is not support; it's shaming, and you have a right to explain that to her. Or if your partner says, "I'm really impressed with the changes you've made in how you eat," thank him or her for being supportive in a way that is helping you to achieve your goals.

Janice—I couldn't have lost thirty pounds in six months without support. One of my daughters was living in the same city as me at the time. She loved to come over on weekends and bake cookies—that was a stress reliever for her. Well, that sure wasn't going to work for me, and when I explained that, she started making soups instead. God bless her—that was support! And she was delighted with the results for herself as well.

Support from Groups and Community Members

Support can be found in many places beyond your family and friends. It might be beneficial for you to consider finding and actively participating in a support group. Researchers have found that successful dieters "emphasized the importance of regular contact in order to maintain motivation and focus on the weight loss goals."[1] The sense of **support** and **accountability** seemed to be the two most important factors. Those who felt positive about being in a group program stressed the importance of belonging to a community that provided opportunities for sharing experiences, motivation, inspiration, as well as problem-solving. "Crucially, the sense of support and accountability was driven not by fear of embarrassment that might be associated with peer pressure, but by feelings of loyalty and obligation to the program leader and the group members."

However, it's possible that when you read the words *support group*, you think you'd just as soon have a root canal. If that's the case, then consider whether having your own accountability partner for support and motivation will help you achieve your goals. Or perhaps you can consider joining an online group. Think about what support looks like to you, write about it, and then get going. You may want to do all of these things or try one and see how it goes.

Janice—Let's be real here. It might not be possible to avoid certain people who are in no way supportive to you as you make these substantive changes. Let me tell you a story:

There was (and is) a person in my life who feels truly toxic for me. It's not just that I don't like them; I don't like myself when I'm interacting with them. I finally realized that I had been mentally concocting a poison to give to that person, but that I had been the one actually drinking it by dwelling in resentment and negativity. Ultimately, I found a way to stop drinking the poison—by which I mean I stopped emotionally engaging, at least when the same old push-button issues were raised. I still don't like them and wish we didn't have to interact so much, but I no longer feel so negatively "attached." They no longer seem to have power over me. I learned that I could change my perception of what had seemed, incorrectly, to be a threat. That person may never change—but I was able to change my response to that person.

In reality, it may be the case that you are not be able to—or do not even want to—eliminate an unsupportive person from your life. The key is to ensure that you have control over your responses to their hurtful words and/or behavior. You can choose to respond with calm and clarity and distance yourself emotionally or physically from the hurtfulness.

Support from Technology—Jae Shares Her Wisdom

Jae—Although it may seem like a paradox, you can use technology to become less *sedentary and* more *socially connected. There are so many resources out there, and these are some of the ones that were integral to my own success. I encourage you to use my suggestions as a starting point. Take the time to do your own research, and feel free to try out other options. You may even discover things I never would have thought of!*

1. Forum Websites

What distinguishes a forum website from a blog or social media page is the idea that you are engaging and interacting with other users. Being part of a supportive and committed community was incredibly helpful and beneficial in helping me to stick with my plans. For many people, support from friends and family is sufficient. For me, though, it was helpful to get support from people who, like me, were also attempting to change their lifestyle and adopt new habits. I learned that when there was someone else to whom I was accountable, I was much more likely to follow through with my plan and make healthy choices. Whenever I accomplished something, like choosing blueberries over a blueberry muffin, these people celebrated with me with a level of understanding that a friend who has never struggled with food or weight would not have been able to understand.

I found this community support in the Reddit forums reddit.com/r/ loseit and reddit.com/r/progresspics. In my opinion, /r/progresspics is a good place to start. People post "before and after" photos (and for most people, it's a work in progress!), and include their height, starting weight, current weight in the "after" photo, and their goal weight. Anyone who goes on the forum is able to find people who are their same height and gender and get a better idea of what they might look like at different stages in their transformation. This was an incredible source of motivation for me, showing me in a real and visible way that what I wanted to do could, in fact, be done.

At the very least, I encourage you to look at the FAQ section for insight into how weight loss works, more detailed descriptions of calorie counting, and other subreddit communities that may be of help to you.

2. MyFitnessPal

MyFitnessPal has been my favorite tool throughout this process; I still use it daily even today. In essence, it is a calorie-counting website and phone app with an extensive and straightforward database of foods to log in their system. This can be extremely helpful in many situations, like when you're at a party or out for dinner and don't have nutrition data available—just type in a food or dish, and you'll get the nutrition information. There's also a great feature where you can log the total ingredients for a dish you're making and how many servings it will be, and the app will automatically calculate the nutrition information per serving. This is super-helpful for people who cook family-sized dishes or who meal prep and cook in bulk (like me). Finally, they have a map and restaurant search feature where you can search the menu of a well-known restaurant and be given nutrition information right within the app.

3. MapMyFitness

MapMyFitness is one of many activity tracking apps for your phone that enables you to calculate your caloric output when you're physically active. One of the things I really like about MapMyFitness is that you can customize it. For example, I have the app set up to announce my time and speed every half mile so I can pace myself and get an idea of how far along I am in my run. The app can do this for all sorts of activities, such as walking, cycling, and hiking.

4. Instagram and Social Media

As time went on, I found that maintenance was going to require an entirely new mindset when it came to my relationship with food and movement. One of the greatest tools for this has been Instagram and, to some extent, Facebook groups. Many Instagram pages provide inspiration regarding meal prep, colorful foods, and nutrition. Some of my favorite accounts are those with beautiful pictures, as well as information about meal prep and nutrition. If you are constantly exposed to positive messages and positive images, it will have a powerful effect on what you take from your news feed. I would caution you to be sure that the accounts you follow are not promoting problematic messages, such as overexercising and unrealistic standards of beauty.

Who supports you in your physical, emotional, and even spiritual life? Think broadly and creatively about who will enhance, rather than undermine, your efforts and intentions. Here is your next list.

List #8: Your Supports

We urge you to identify sources of support and ask for what you need. Please keep in mind that in so doing, you're showing signs of strength, not weakness. As the saying goes: "a self-made man is like a self-laid egg."

CHAPTER 13

From Bad Habits to Brilliant Strategies

> Perhaps the most important habit to change is the habit of saying negative things to yourself about yourself.

Janice—Here's a daily snapshot of my old life: I come home from work and automatically walk straight to the refrigerator. Am I hungry? I doubt it; I wasn't even thinking about food two minutes ago. But here I am with a fork in my hand, stabbing at random items. Here's another snapshot from that life: I've had dinner, and I'm now in my den, reading or watching television. There's a plate of cookies next to me. Or there was—I hardly remember eating them at all.

Do you have mindless eating-related habits, too? Especially when your brain is overwhelmed by stress, anxiety, sadness, and other negative emotions, one of its likely responses is to go numb. Here's what might happen:

- Whenever you go for a coffee break at work or between classes, you always automatically include a quick stop for a donut and a chocolate caramel double latte.

- Clearing plates from the table means that you also unthinkingly finish off what's left on your kids' plates while you walk over to the sink.
- You have a bowl of chips in your lap while you're watching television. Suddenly, you look down at the empty bowl and wonder, how is that possible?

Notice that in all the examples above, we're talking about ingrained, automatic **habits**. You simply go on autopilot without thinking about how or why the behavior even happens.

How Habits Form

Here's how habits develop: you know from past experience that eating a cookie (or six) will soothe your sadness, bad mood, anger, frustration, stress, or boredom, at least temporarily. After you've done this enough times, the emotional component doesn't even need to be there; eating the cookie becomes increasingly automatic. That's how habits develop—when a recurring situation leads to a recurring behavior, omitting a rational thought process between the two. There have been plenty of studies that bear this out and show that obesity is associated with automatic or impulsive behavior.[1, 2] Honestly, though, did you really need studies to prove that?

Jae—Mindless eating, not just eating junk food, was such a bad habit for me. In high school, my schedule was incredibly packed, and I was often traveling to and from school, extracurricular activities, and my job. I used to keep cereal and other snacks in the back seat of my car and eat them by the handful. Was I aware of how much I was eating? Of course not. I was just shoveling it in while I drove! I don't keep food in the car anymore. I don't want to eat unless I'm feeling in control.

It's hard to change habits. It's hard to try something new when you enjoy—or are at least accustomed to—the way things are now. Remember, though, that habits are not commands. They are bundled behaviors that get repeated until they become automatic. Breaking a habit is hard, but it is certainly possible. What we propose is, first of all, to replace the "automatic" part of the habit with **conscious, deliberate thought**. Do you *have* to respond in the same way to a situation that you always have? You probably don't. Think about your routines—what you do when you get up each morning, what your work or study breaks look like, what you prepare or buy for meals, what you do when you get home, or how you spend your relaxation time. Once you're aware of how a routine has morphed into a destructive habit, then you can replace the unwanted habit with a new one. This actually works—we swear! The original habit truly does become remarkably less powerful over time as the new, healthier habit gets repeated.

Identify and Replace

What we propose is to first of all, **identify** your current habits. Think about what you're doing and whether you have to respond in the same way that you always have. There's a good chance that you don't. What are the habits you would like to change? What are possible remedies?

Second of all, **replace** one habit with another. Here are some examples:

- You get home at the end of the day, and instead of plopping down in front of your computer screen with a glass of wine, grab an apple and eat it while you're putting on your work-out clothes. And then work out, of course.

- Before the Netflix marathon starts, instead of getting out the chips, get some cherries and carrot sticks—because aside from fruit or vegetables, the den is now a food-free zone.

- You no longer wake up, roll over, and scroll through Facebook for twenty minutes. Instead, take a twenty-minute brisk walk. Beginning your morning with movement and fresh air can be an energizing way to start your day. Tell the truth: do you feel energized after scrolling through Facebook?

- Your daily coffee break no longer consists of a donut in the coffee room or a pastry from the coffee shop. Instead, you've brought yogurt and fruit or a handful of nuts. Enjoy your coffee and the healthy snack that you've planned for—and you remember to congratulate yourself. Repeat. Daily.

- You step in front of the mirror, and your Evil Twin starts reciting the usual negative list of what's wrong with you. Instead of letting these self-defeating, untrue thoughts take over the space in your brain, make the conscious decision to stop the script and reframe the thoughts into something positive.

You'll notice that almost all of these healthy habits have to do with **stimulus control**. You no longer put unhealthy, impossible-to-resist foods in front of you because doing so simply isn't fair to yourself. In a study on the behavioral treatment of obesity, the authors found that the key elements of treatment included goal setting and stimulus control. This is what helps us to "change the internal and external cues" associated with problem eating and behavior.[3]

This is a good time for your next list.

List #9: Out with the Old, In with the New

On one side, write down an old habit. On the other side, write down how you can eliminate or replace that habit. Keep going!

Bundle Up

You'll also notice that by bundling two activities in a new way, you're reinforcing, creating, and sustaining new habits. Each time you do this, the connection strengthens.

Janice—Years ago, I took up needlepoint and knitting to help me stop smoking. Now, I find those activities really useful in breaking the repetitive hand-in-the-bowl syndrome when I'm watching television. Another example is from one of my patients, who told me she hadn't cooked for herself because she hated food shopping. She then chose a yoga class specifically because the studio was near a grocery store she liked, and she got in the habit of going to the store after every yoga class.

Jae—When I used to go to the movies, I'd go all out and buy my favorite things—buttered popcorn, chocolate, and maybe some other candy. I would tell myself that it was okay to buy all three things because I would share them with my friends and would be able to have self-control. Then we'd start watching the movie, and I would be so engrossed in it that I wouldn't even realize I'd eaten everything myself! Finally, I would feel ashamed and disappointed in myself.

Now when I go to the movies, if I take anything at all, I take a bag of carrots. Carrots are crunchy, and they keep my mouth and hands busy just like chips or popcorn would. If I want something sweet, then I take grapes. Because I've planned ahead, I'm no longer mindlessly eating junk while paying attention to something else.

Janice—*I have a question: What is it about food and movies? When you go to a play, you don't eat while you're watching. When you go to a concert, you don't eat while you're listening. But when you go to the movies, it seems perfectly normal to get a bucket of popcorn the size of an actual bucket and a soda that would suffice for a trek across a desert. What on earth is that about?*

Everyone Slips Up Sometimes

While you're working toward breaking these ingrained habits, you might find yourself slipping up. Don't worry about it—it's okay. Slipups are part of the process; they do *not* represent failure. Don't let the mistake derail you from your long-term goals; stay on track and continue to think about the big picture.

Janice—*A very tough habit to break for me is when I really, really want something sweet after I eat. Now I have a bunch of grapes or some berries next to the dinner plate to snack on. I then immediately brush my teeth. I also make every attempt to leave the kitchen once dinner is over. But honestly? Once in a while, it just doesn't work. I'll admit it: I have a stash of sugar-free hard candy, and sometimes I'll have one. I don't like this candy very much, so I'm able to limit myself to one. Yes, it's garbage; yes, it upsets my stomach; and yes, it makes it harder to get past my craving for sweets. But there it is. I am so not perfect—I'm still a work in progress.*

Too Much Structure?

Perhaps you're put off by what sounds like too much structure to the point of rigidity. Will you have to live such a structured life forever? We can't answer that question. We can tell you, though, that the two of us are still very structured with regard to what we eat and how we eat. But we don't view this as a burden—in fact, it's quite the opposite. This structure is a relief from the chaos of crazy eating followed by self-recrimination. It's a way of taking care of ourselves and of maintaining calm. And think about it—aren't damaging habits structured and rigid, too? Habits are, in essence, routines that separate thought and action so you can function more efficiently—at least that's what they should be. Take control of these automatic responses so that they become tools you can rely on for reaching your goals.

Perhaps the most important habit to change is the habit of saying negative things to yourself about yourself. Try to catch yourself every time this happens—replace the script with something positive and kind. This change, while the most important, may also be the most difficult—you've had a lifetime to perfect the practice of negative thoughts and self-talk. But positivity becomes such a motivator, and it's worth the effort. In fact, if you can change just this one habit, then we can confidently offer you the promise of a happier, fuller, richer life.

STEP SIX:

Make Your Brain Your Greatest Ally

CHAPTER 14

Eating Your Feelings—
a Recipe for Failure

When you eat a single piece of chocolate, do you feel like a shark tasting blood?

You walk into your house, exhausted and angry. Your bus never showed up. You're cold, and your feet hurt. You open the refrigerator and see a bag of carrots and a leftover slice of pizza. Guess which one you're more likely to reach for? We get it—you're stressed, physically and emotionally. You want relief. Pizza seems like a good idea.

Stress is a negative emotional and physical experience that often has behavioral consequences. Stress eating is one of those consequences (and, as we'll explain soon, a *cause* of emotional stress as well). Stress eating is real, and it's a powerful, commonly used type of emotional reward. It surely comes as no surprise to you that stress eaters typically don't crave celery; they're "much more likely to crave high-fat/sweet and rewarding comfort foods."[1]

A No-Win Situation

Unfortunately, what happens is most people who eat to alleviate stress actually feel *more* stressed after they eat in an unhealthy way.[2]

Not only that, but foods rich in sugar may actually increase hunger signals and decrease fullness signals in the brain.[3] In other words, as we've talked about earlier in Chapter 7, using food as a way to calm or soothe yourself has one major problem: it doesn't work. It may feel like a solution at the time, but the temporary fix is not only short-lived, but also almost invariably followed by remorse and even shame.

Acute stress is associated with increased eating, particularly "palatable, calorie-dense" food.[4, 5] That may seem obvious to you. But what is less obvious, and is much more insidious and dangerous, is how *chronic* stress affects both physical and mental health.

The way chronic stress is associated with weight gain[6, 7] is related to how reward centers in the brain are activated and how stress hormones (especially cortisol) increase and then change appetite-regulating hormones (such as insulin, leptin, and ghrelin).[8] These chemicals also increase the brain and body's desire for highly palatable foods,[9] even when you're not physically hungry. As a result, stress responses then become increasingly powerful and ingrained habits. MRI studies have shown that chronic stress activates the reward centers of the brain and deactivates the parts of the brain associated with planning and emotional control.[10]

As we've emphasized throughout this book, desire for food that is detached from physical hunger leads to a type of eating response that is ultimately self-defeating. Even being "on a diet" is stressful enough to lead some people to desire food more than they would have otherwise! What is more, the increase in the stress hormone cortisol is associated with an increased risk of abdominal obesity, metabolic syndrome, cardiovascular disease, and type 2 diabetes.[11] Children are also vulnerable to these very same risks.[12]

Food Cues: The Start of Trouble

In Chapter 9, we talked about food cues in our discussion of trigger foods. A food cue is a particular food, a picture of a food (particularly in advertisements), or the aroma of a food that makes you "hungry" for that food, even if your body isn't actually physically hungry.[13, 14, 15] In this way, food cues act very much in the way that stress does. And like stress-related responses, food cues are learned, conditioned responses that create a strong desire and are associated with weight gain.[16] This is true for children, as well as adults.[17] Chronic stress is a major factor in leading a food cue to spark the sensation of craving, defined as "an intense desire or urge to eat" a particular food."[18] Let's sort that out.

Craving: More than Just Wanting

How many of us have found ourselves at a convenience store at some ungodly hour of the night and literally *prayed* that no one we knew would see us? Because if they actually did see us, then we'd have to make up an excuse and walk out with a bottle of Tylenol instead of a family-size bag of M&M's? When you eat a single piece of chocolate, do you feel like a shark tasting blood? Does that single piece just make you want to have twenty more? We feel your pain. We have *experienced* your pain.

The brain reacts to the sight and smell of tasty food. That's a normal response. But for some people, the brain's response goes way beyond "normal." Stress makes your cravings stronger and increases your sense of feeling out of control. Cravings aren't the same as hunger. If you're hungry, then an apple is just fine. A craving, on the other hand, can eradicate rational thinking and is almost always for a specific food that is "a highly processed food that contains lots of refined carbohydrates and fat."[19] How many times have you heard someone say, "Man, I'm really dying for a cucumber"? We're going to guess never.

Jae—When I start eating food that has high added sugar content, I just want more and more. I keep craving it. I can't get it out of my head, and then I naturally gravitate toward sugary foods for the rest of the day. In fact, early on in the process of losing weight, I cut out processed sugary foods almost completely—it was my sugar detox. Even now, I know I need to be mindful of how and when I choose to eat processed sweet foods.

It isn't fair, but overweight people tend to experience more intense cravings. MRI studies make clear that this is partially because overweight people have a greater "reward region" in the brain that makes them more responsive to crave-worthy foods.[20] *Cravings are not your fault!* However, since you're a grown-up, you're nonetheless responsible for dealing with them, and we promise to help.

Craving or Addiction? Can a Single French Fry Be a Gateway Drug?

For some people, certain foods, particularly highly processed ones like ice cream, chocolate, pizza, French fries, and soda, may trigger an addictive-type response.[21] Just as with addictive drugs, highly palatable foods trigger chemicals in the brain's reward pathway and lead to the drive to eat even more of those foods. Yes, just like a shark tasting blood.

Jae—Alcoholics do not need alcohol to survive. Smokers do not need cigarettes to survive. Alcohol and tobacco are not biologically necessary nutrients, and their absence is not fatal. It's different with food! This sounds silly, but what if you feel addicted to food? You do *have to eat to survive. It's hard to constantly face this anxiety about food and food choices.*

So, what's a person to do? Feeling like a slave to cravings is emotionally and physically unhealthy. It's horrible to feel so out of control. Even if you're not "addicted," the connection between feeling stressed and using food to relieve stress is *powerful*. That's why change is difficult! Can you learn skills to cope with stress in a way that is helpful rather than destructive? The answer is a definite *yes*—you can actually train your brain to be more resilient, more adaptable, and able to manage stress more effectively. You can define and implement your own techniques to diminish the effects of stressful thoughts and situations. Please turn the page.

CHAPTER 15

Stress Relief, Part 1—Leave Your Lizard Brain Behind

Mindfulness will be your best friend when you're trying to cope with stress and its associated miseries, including emotional eating.

Slow It Down. Way Down.

Here's an emergency: you're in the jungle, and you see a tiger. Obviously, you're not going to stop and think, "Hmm, big animal with orange and black stripes, sharp claws, huge teeth . . ." If you take the time to do that, you're going to be lunch for that tiger. Deliberate, considered thought is *not* what you need when a stressful situation is a true emergency. Rather, you need to use a more primitive part of your brain that developed early during evolution—your *lizard brain*, as it's often called—to respond quickly to danger. Your lizard brain will then put you in fight-or-flight mode, rather than the think-deeply-about-your-options mode. In the tiger situation, the latter is sure to end badly.

The decision about what to eat, on the other hand, is *not* an emergency. The decision about how to deal with an unpleasant person or situation is *not* an emergency. The decision about how to respond to a sad day is *not* an emergency. These are circumstances where you want to use the thinking and reasoning part of your brain—your cerebral cortex—and leave the lizard brain behind. But when you're stressed or anxious, everything speeds up, and not in a good way. You move fast—but in circles. You think fast—but not clearly. There's even evidence that the part of your brain that intentionally speeds up—i.e., multitasking—may not always be efficient and may also result in increased anxiety and stress.[1]

In contrast, when you slow down your thoughts in response to a stressful situation, you can make the shift from **reacting** to **responding**. **Reaction** is immediate, urgent, and less thought out. When there is no pause after a stimulus, you react with the primitive lizard brain, the part that acts first and thinks later. **Response**, on the other hand, is slower, more thoughtful, and makes use of your cognitive powers.

Everyone experiences stress. Psychological stress occurs when something uncomfortable happens that requires you to respond in a way that restores equilibrium to your brain. Again, the key word here is *respond*. Responding, as opposed to reacting, is a slowing down, a pause, a space.

Viktor Frankl, the great writer, psychiatrist, and Holocaust survivor, put it best: "Between stimulus and response, there is a space. In that space is our power to choose our response. In our response lies our growth and our freedom."

For the two of us, **slowing down to think about our choices and their consequences** has been, in many ways, the single most important element of our weight loss success. This success applies to both sustaining our weight loss, and, more important, to becoming happier, calmer, and more effective people.

It's common for people to react to a stressful situation in a way that doesn't allow the brain to "let go" of the stress. Negative emotions, such as anxiety and anger, can overwhelm your ability to move past the situation, even when the situation has passed. Not surprisingly, stress is one of the major barriers to successful, sustainable weight loss.[2] In this chapter and the next, we're going to show you how you can respond more effectively when stressful situations arise and, specifically, how you can conquer emotional overeating as a response to stress.

There are plenty of *big* stresses for all of us—loss of a loved one, the end of a relationship, illness, and financial stress, to name a few. Even happy times can be really stressful—a wedding, a new baby, or a new job, for example. But it's *little* stresses that can make us chronically irritable and anxious—the cashier who seems to smirk a tiny bit as she puts up the "next lane please" card just as you arrive with your grocery cart, or the jerk who won't let you change traffic lanes, perhaps because his very manhood is at stake. These *minor* stresses can be *major* contributors to unhappiness if you're not able to respond to them in a way that doesn't eat you alive.

The good news is you can actually choose how you want to respond in these situations. Do you want to fume and become increasingly enraged as you consider your choice of verbal weapons, or would you rather just shrug your shoulders and think about something pleasant? Perhaps you might even want to envision a scenario that reframes the entire situation. Did the cashier's boyfriend just break up with her? Is the guy in the car driving to the hospital because his child was in an accident? Who knows? The point is, you may not be able to control the stressor, but there's a good chance you can control your response.

Janice—*I can't always trust myself to envision these scenarios of compassion. This is why I always bring a book into the grocery store in case there is a long line and why I leave a little early for work so I don't go crazy in traffic. It's also why I don't stress myself by having cookies in the house or seeking out all-you-can-eat buffets. I do what I can to minimize stress in a way that doesn't cause* distress *to myself (or anyone else, for that matter—because I really am tempted to gesture angrily to that guy in the car next to me).*

Mindfulness: Increasing the Space between Stimulus and Response

What might it look like if you could increase that space between the stimulus and your response? It could look like considering options. It could look like being less defensive, less judgmental, and more attentive. It would look like slowing down and thinking calmly, which is the exact opposite of fight-or-flight action,[3] an action that is driven by a sense of urgency or even panic.

There's been so much written about that mind-numbingly over-used word *mindfulness* that it's become a cliché. There's a reason for that, though. Mindfulness will be your best friend when you're trying to cope with stress and its associated miseries, including emotional eating. Mindfulness affords you a pause, an opportunity for awareness. In other words, mindfulness is **paying attention**. Jon Kabat-Zinn, the pioneer in the mindfulness-based stress reduction movement, describes mindfulness as "the awareness that arises from paying attention on purpose, in the present moment, nonjudgmentally."[4] What is the result of that focused attention? Increased clarity, resilience, and peace of mind.

Don't Believe Everything You Think

In Chapter 3, we talked about paving the path from thoughts to action in order to achieve a desired outcome. Thoughts truly are important, but they're not everything that goes on in your brain. Let us explain.

Thoughts are just that. They're not facts. They're not truths. Mindfulness provides a means for looking at situations more objectively and creatively. Stress can have a lasting—and distorted—effect on thoughts. It activates areas of the brain that control anxiety and other negative emotions. It leads you to think that your current unhappy feelings will last forever. It leads you to think that the bad things you've invented about yourself are factual. Stress is a powerful ally of your Evil Twin that we talked about in Chapter 3.

Mindfulness, on the other hand, improves psychological well-being by enabling you to evaluate situations and feel emotions in a more accepting and less judgmental, critical way. It helps you view a stressor as a signal, not an order. A study showed that mindfulness training leads to a faster recovery from emotions such as sadness and anger.[5]

You're in Control

It is also known that major barriers to long-term weight loss include **reward-driven eating**, which is characterized by a lack of control over eating and a preoccupation with food, as well as **psychological stress.** Mindfulness training may address these barriers and promote weight loss by reducing stress and increasing awareness of hunger and fullness cues. Consider this example:

"I'm starving! I have to eat this bag of chips right now!" Believe us, we know this feeling. You *need* these chips—immediately. Your diet doesn't matter, your health doesn't matter, your promises to yourself don't matter. The chips matter.

But hold on a second. Your health and your promises to yourself *do* matter, and you know they do—five minutes after you polish off the chips, you're going to think about how you let yourself down by abandoning your intentions to eat in a healthier way. You were in that state of feeling so out of control and thinking that you had to have the chips, but that wasn't the way it had to be. You actually *are* in control, you *do* have a choice, and you can choose to respond differently. You can choose to challenge your thoughts and pause long enough to remind yourself that you actually do not *have* to have the chips. You can walk away from them, literally or metaphorically, and do something else. And, of course, congratulate yourself when you do that.

You Can Train Your Brain

Mindfulness meditation, as a form of mindfulness training, has been shown to stimulate areas of the brain that control mood, emotional eating, problem-solving ability, and self-control.[6, 7] All of these qualities work together to help decrease depression and enable you to be more resilient to stress.[8] Meditation has been shown to be not just a stress *reliever*, but also a stress *preventer*.

This is how Jon Kabat-Zinn describes mindfulness meditation: "Feel a breath come in and feel a breath go out, attending only to the breath itself. But inevitably, perhaps even very rapidly, you begin to notice your mind drifting off to something else . . . bring your attention back to your breathing—it's like exercising a muscle: the mind goes off, you bring it back, the mind goes off, you bring it back . . ."

Using MRI scans, researchers showed that after just eight weeks of beginning a daily meditation practice, there was an increased amount of gray matter in areas of the brain associated with memory and emotional regulation.[9] Think about it: meditation actually changes the very *structure* of the brain!

Janice—For me, practicing meditation daily, even if it's only for a few minutes some days, has decreased my anxiety and made it possible to *access a mental space of relaxation. More than that, I can now access that calm space even when I'm not meditating.*

Jae—*While I don't meditate, I certainly identify with the idea of decreasing anxiety. It's such a common feeling when it comes to food. We all need to find an outlet for this. We all need to find some way to feel in control. For me, my outlets are going for a walk, which calms me down and also gives me the chance to find new things in the city; and coloring—there's something so satisfying about filling in a geometric design exactly all the way throughout the whole picture. Very zen.*

If you remain unconvinced about meditation, that's just fine. There are lots of ways to slow down your brain. At the very least, try this and see how it feels:

Find a comfortable spot to sit. Set a timer for three minutes (or, if you worry that waiting for it to go off will make you anxious, just estimate three minutes and check the clock when you think it's time—no big deal). Close your eyes, and pay attention to your breath. Breathe in, breathe out. That's it. When thoughts float through, which of course they will, just return to the breath.

When the timer goes off, notice how you feel. We think you'll be astonished by how rested and refreshed you feel after a mere three minutes.

Challenge False Ideas about Failure

Throughout this book, we've emphasized that slipups are part of the process of change. Perhaps you're eating ice cream by the pint or your sneakers have begun to gather dust. Being aware—and even accepting—of these setbacks will help you move forward instead of getting stuck in a mire of self-recrimination.

Don't let a setback allow you to doubt your ability to choose a healthier life for yourself. Challenge the thought that since diets haven't worked before, then the changes you're making now probably won't work either. Challenge other people's "advice" if it's hurtful to you. Remember, you're choosing to respond, not just react. Taking that little bit of extra time affords you the opportunity to question long-held, but untrue, self-critical accusations. Take the time to change the script! You already know that feeling guilty or angry with yourself doesn't work, right? So why not try something else that has evidence behind it?

Another wretchedly overused phrase is "living in the moment." Again, however, the reason it's a cliché is that there's so much truth to it. You can't change the past, nor can you know the future. The present is all there is, and paying close attention to it, with as little judgment as possible, is a rewarding way to live. The *process* is the reward.

CHAPTER 16

Stress Relief, Part 2— You're Getting Sleepy

> Sleep-deprived people eat more food; they eat more frequently; and they tend to eat late at night.

In the previous chapter, we talked about mindfulness as a tool to help you pay close attention and increase the space between stimulus and response. This is the key to changing out-of-control eating habits to a deeply satisfying enjoyment of food and your body. Now we'll give you other tools to add to your collection, starting with that most magical of phenomena, sleep.

Sleep Is Not a Luxury

We're putting sleep at the top of the toolbox list because there's a good chance that you, like most Americans, don't get enough sleep; and because sleep is an essential, non-negotiable component of sustainable weight loss (along with physical and emotional health).

Janice—Take it from me, an obstetrician: you may be able to train your brain and body to function on inadequate sleep, at least temporarily, but you can't train your brain and body to need *less sleep. You need what you need.*

Almost one-third of Americans get fewer than six hours of sleep a night.[1] Sleep-deprived people eat more food; they eat more frequently; and they tend to eat late at night, a time when they're likely to eat higher-calorie food. In fact, sleep-deprived people eat an average of 300 to 550 calories more per day than people who get adequate sleep (approximately eight hours per night).[2] Do the math: that adds up to between 30 and 57 pounds a year if they kept that up every day!

Why does this happen? Why are sleep and eating habits so inter-connected? One major reason is that when you're sleep-deprived, both your body's hormones and your brain's response to food change in a way to make you hungrier, especially for foods high in sugar, fat, and salt.[3, 4] The result is that if you're chronically sleep-deprived, you're at a much greater risk for obesity and its complications, such as diabetes and heart disease.[5, 6] The reverse is true as well: just as inadequate sleep increases the risk for obesity, the presence of obesity impairs sleep. [7, 8] This is even true for children.[9]

It's not just appetite and weight that are affected, either. Here are four other very predictable consequences if you regularly get too little sleep:

1. Your mood is affected—and never in a good way. You become more irritable and more likely to be depressed.[10]
2. You don't think or concentrate as well. And because your judgment is impaired, you're not even aware that you're not as sharp.[11]
3. Your immune system becomes weaker, leaving you more sus-ceptible to illness and even earlier death.[12]

4. You are more likely to cause and/or be a victim of a serious injury, particularly a car crash.[13, 14]

Janice—Let me tell you about my favorite, if unnecessary, study.[15] I'm sure you're aware of the common wisdom that you shouldn't go food shopping when you're tired or hungry. Well, there's scientific proof that the common wisdom is correct. Researchers gave two groups of men, one sleep-deprived and one not, money to buy food at the grocery store. The sleep-deprived men bought more food and more high-calorie, unhealthy food than the men who'd gotten enough sleep.

In summary, if you think you're saving time by sleeping less, then think again. You'll be grumpy, you won't think well, and you'll be more vulnerable to sickness and injury. And please don't kid yourself when you say you can "catch up" on sleep on the weekends or whenever—that strategy simply doesn't work.

Janice—As one of my patients put it, "Routine is important to me now. On weekends, I used to sleep in really late. Then, when I got up, I munched a little here and there. I would eat and eat and eat and still feel hungry. And somehow, I'd still be famished by dinner."

Circadian Rhythm & Blues

We realize that some of this may be out of your control, especially if your circadian rhythm is all messed up by working nontraditional hours, traveling across time zones, or staying up with a crying baby.[16] Just know that you're paying a price. Normally, there is synchrony in how the brain responds to light, sleep, and eating rhythms over a twenty-four-hour period—that's what circadian rhythm means. Disrupting this normal rhythm with too little sleep or irregular sleep takes a big toll on your brain and body, including putting you at an increased risk for diabetes and heart disease.[17, 18] Even your gut microbiome responds to circadian rhythms![19]

Jae—During high school, I was incredibly busy with school, extracurricular, activities, and just being a teenager. There were days when I got up at 5:30 a.m. and came home at 10 p.m., only to stay up until midnight studying. Along with using food as a coping mechanism for emotional stress, I'm sure sleeping five hours a night added to the twenty pounds a year I was gaining in high school.

Once I got to college, I found a routine that worked for me—one that included a lot *of sleep. I still make sure I get a minimum of seven hours a night or usually more. I live my best life when I'm getting eight hours of sleep. This is so important to me because I can feel how it affects my mood, my hunger, and my approach to food. I'm more patient, and I can think more clearly—not to mention I have so much more energy.*

So our take-home message is this: do your best to live and work in such a way that you can sleep for eight hours every night, and preferably go to bed around the same time every night so your body can get used to the routine. Do whatever you can to have fun and joy in your life, but make a sincere commitment to get the sleep you need, not the sleep you think you have time for.

A Daytime Nap: The Pause That Refreshes

If you can't get enough sleep at night, then short naps during the day may be just the thing for you. That's assuming you get six hours of sleep a night at the very least. If you do, then short naps may dramatically increase your alertness.[20] For most people, a ten-minute nap is ideal with regard to minimal post-sleep grogginess and maximal post-sleep alertness. These short naps enhance working memory, emotional regulation, and learning ability.[21]

Time to Reboot!

Here's some really good news: overweight people who increased their sleeping time from under six and a half hours per night to seven to nine hours per night for just two weeks not only felt less tired and more energetic, but also experienced a 14 percent decrease in appetite, mostly due to a decreased craving for sweets and salty food.[22] There's even more good news: once you do lose weight, you're likely to sleep much better because of the potential for resolution of sleep apnea[23] and general body discomfort. Nighty-night.

CHAPTER 17

Stress Relief, Part 3— Putting It Together

> There is an enormous difference between saying, "I can't eat this," and saying, "I'm choosing not to eat this."

Now it's time to talk about applying stress management techniques to specific eating-related issues. We have found these to be of great value in our ongoing positive relationship with food. Adapt them as you like, and develop strategies of your own.

Mindful Eating: The Magic Raisin

Perhaps you've heard of the raisin exercise. It sounds really hokey—in fact, it *is* really hokey. But it's also amazing. Here's what it is:

You're given a single raisin and told not to eat it. Just look at it, notice the shape, the wrinkles, the color. Notice how it feels in your hand. Think about what it might taste like, but don't put it in your mouth yet. After a minute or two of this, you're told to put the raisin in your mouth, but not to bite down on it. Simply feel the texture of it on your tongue and that sort of thing. Finally, after what feels like an eternity (it's actually about three minutes or so), you're told you can bite down on the raisin, chew it slowly, and swallow it.

Here's what most people experience: the raisin absolutely explodes with flavor. It's the most incredible, delicious thing you've ever tasted in your life. You know that's ridiculous—it's a raisin, for goodness sake—but still, your mouth feels overwhelmed by the wonderful taste. We are not suggesting that you eat all your food like this all the time. However, we hope that we've made a good enough case for mindfulness that you'll want to apply those strategies of awareness and presence toward how you eat.

Savor your food. How do you do that? We'll tell you what works, but first we'll mention what's guaranteed *not* to work: we promise you will be unable to savor food if you're eating something you think you shouldn't be eating but that you want anyway; you know you'll be sorry afterward, but right now you just can't help yourself—whew! Forget that. Throughout this book, we've stressed the importance of taking time to make good decisions for yourself, planning what you're going to eat ahead of time, and setting yourself up for success. If you plan what you're going to eat, and that's exactly what you put on the table, then you really *can* savor your food! You can enjoy every single bite.

Speaking of bites, we recommend that you take small bites. Put down the fork between each bite, and chew and swallow your food before the next. No, it's not going to be a raisin experience every time you eat, but this method allows you to eat slowly and intentionally. Eating more slowly and in a more relaxed, mindful state has been shown to result in significantly more controlled eating.[1, 2] A major reason for this is it gives your brain more time (it usually takes about twenty minutes) to register fullness. Slower, more mindful eating provides your brain and body with an opportunity to have a dialogue with each other. You'll be able to recognize fullness cues better, you'll be able to make better food choices, and you don't have to sneak food into your mouth.

Meditation in Aisle 6

It might not be a meditative experience, but grocery shopping should certainly be a mindful one. Make a list ahead of time (planning is your best friend in the world), and stick to the list. If you've got apples on the list, don't kid yourself into making a "swap" for an apple pie. Impulse buying is the work of the devil. Throughout this book, we've talked about trigger foods (Chapter 9), food cues (Chapter 14), and setting yourself up for success (Chapter 11). If you live with someone who is trying to stop drinking alcohol or quit smoking, you wouldn't go out and buy a bottle of vodka or a carton of cigarettes, and tell your partner to "just say no"—that's not fair. So, don't do it to yourself, either. Make your home a safe space for yourself.

Let's suppose, though, that after you've put the apples in your grocery cart, you also add the apple pie "in case I have company." Then, after you've been home for a while, you get hungry and want a snack. For most of us, it's really hard to choose the apple. Here's what to do: *pause*. Slow it down. Stop and think. Use your mindfulness tools from Chapter 15. How will you feel about yourself in five minutes if you eat the pie? What about the apple? How about tomorrow? Let me tell you, you're going to feel proud of yourself for eating the apple. You're going to have that confidence that comes with being in control, and you can build on that. All from eating one apple!

Janice—Having said that, as I write all these encouraging words about choosing the apple, I know full well that if there was a pie in my house, there might not be any pie left tomorrow. I know myself. That's why choosing not to have any pies at home at all works for me.

End the Deprivation Mindset

You may choose to think about the long-term *costs* of eating unhealthy food in an unhealthy way, or you may decide to focus on the long-term *benefits* of *not* eating that food. Both of those strategies work, but which is best? The answer is the second one: focusing on *benefits*.[3] It's what we've said all along—when you switch from thinking positively about taking care of yourself instead of thinking negatively about deprivation, you're more likely to achieve success. And now there are studies of the brain to prove it. Responding to stress with a considered, conscious choice is an essential paradigm shift in the process of moving away from a deprivation mindset. It will help you feel in charge and competent.

There is an enormous difference between saying, "I can't eat this," and saying, "I'm choosing not to eat this." Don't be derailed by your Evil Twin telling you that eating the apple means that, for the rest of your life, you're stuck with only apples and can never have apple pie again. That's simply not true. Right now, you're just choosing the apple because that's the choice you *want* to make to feel good about yourself in the short term, and it's the choice you want to build on so you'll feel good physically and mentally in the long term. You can always choose to have a slice of pie some other time if that's what you want. Don't turn this into a pity party. *Visualize* how it will feel when your body is no longer at constant war with food.

You Can Change What You Want to Eat!

MRI studies have shown that with time, particularly as you focus on the *benefits* and *value* of your eating changes, your brain will actually adapt in a way that decreases your cravings for unhealthy foods.[4, 5] Think about it: this is literally strength training for the brain—no barbells required! How cool is that?

Learning to Drive

Having said all this, we really do understand that sometimes you just want to wolf down a cheeseburger, and all this healthy-eating stuff starts to feel pretty hollow. Again, this is where practicing mindfulness can be a tremendous ally in helping you to tolerate feelings of discomfort more effectively.

The first time you got behind the wheel of a car, it was probably a miracle that you didn't crash. You thought you'd never learn how to do it. But you did. You practiced, and you learned. A mindful way of life takes time, too. And it will be even more freeing than being able to drive yourself around!

There's one more really, really important piece of the stress management puzzle, and it deserves its own chapter. It's something that will relieve stress, improve your physical and mental health, help you lose weight, and be an essential part of not gaining back the weight you lose. It's called exercise. Please don't slam this book shut now. Trust us. Turn the page.

STEP SEVEN:

Physical Exercise: You Want to Do This. Really.

CHAPTER 18

Physical Activity, Part 1—The Most Important Prescription You Can Ever Fill

> After weight loss, physical activity
> is a major determinant in the
> prevention of future weight gain.

When your doctor gives you a prescription, you are told about the side effects, allergic reactions, and potential risks associated with that medicine. Then, your pharmacist will tell you the cost—after which you may need another prescription for your heart palpitations. How about a prescription for something that will help you feel better, live longer, and live happier; that has few risks and side effects; and that is free? It's called exercise.

Wait! Hear us out! Aside from the incredible physical and mental benefits of physical activity,[1] perhaps its greatest benefit is that it will make you happier. Guaranteed. And now for the details.

Your Body Will Thank You

1. Protection against Heart Disease and Heart Failure

Physical activity protects against the occurrence of heart disease and heart failure, along with death from these diseases.[2] Even as little as twenty minutes a day of brisk walking makes a big difference![3]

2. Protection against Cancer

Physical activity has been shown to lower the risk of more than a dozen different forms of cancer, including breast cancer and colon cancer.[4, 5, 6] Exercise might even help prevent cancer recurrence.[7]

3. Stronger Immune System

Physical activity even increases the diversity of the intestinal microbiome,[8] which, as we talked about in Chapter 4, affects virtually every aspect of the health of your body, including your immune system.

4. Healthier Bones & Joints

Exercise can help prevent knee osteoarthritis and postmenopausal bone loss.[9, 10] Weight-bearing exercise helps to prevent and improve osteoporosis[11] *and to prevent dangerous falls.*[12]

Your Happier, Fitter Brain Will Thank You

Exercise is one of the most effective ways to increase brain function in both younger[13] and older people. It also helps lower the risk of cognitive decline and dementia—even Alzheimer's disease—in later life.[14] In addition to improving the brain's cognitive power, exercise also improves mood and decreases depression in people from their youth to old age.[15, 16, 17]

In other words, if you're between the ages of six and ninety-six, rest assured that exercise will improve your physical health, your brain function, and your mood. And if you have children, your kids are a lot more likely to be physically active if you are, too.

Jae—I love to run because I feel accomplished, physically tough, and mentally strong. Exercise relieves my stress and helps combat my depression more so than any pill has ever done.

When I moved to a new city after I finished college, I loved walking around different neighborhoods as a way to learn about my new home. Also, I walked to and from work, which gave me time to decompress and think—or not think—about all of the things that I had to do!

You'll Enhance Your Weight Loss Progress

The mood-enhancing power of regular exercise is one of the reasons, aside from burning calories, that helps with weight loss. When your overall mood is improved, there is less stress associated with the challenges of changing your relationship with food.[18]

Regular physical activity in childhood and adolescence plays a major *prevention* role[19] against obesity in young adulthood;[20] and young adults who exercise are much less likely to experience the weight gain that is so typical in middle age, particularly in women.[21]

There's a sad truth that once you've lost weight, it becomes harder to lose more. Why? Because your slimmer body needs less fuel to keep it going, which means you need to eat less. But you're already eating so much less! What's the solution to revving up your metabolism? The answer is more exercise. In fact, after weight loss, physical activity is a major determinant in the prevention of future weight gain.[22]

You're Never Too Old for Physical Activity

Exercise is wonderful for older people. Period. We're not talking about getting in shape so that you can wear a bikini again or have six-pack abs. Really, who cares? We're not even talking about living longer (although people who are active do, in fact, live longer).[23] Rather, we're talking about living *better*.[24, 25] The term *physical fitness* refers to "the ability to carry out daily tasks with vigor and alertness without undue fatigue, and with ample energy to enjoy leisure time pursuits and meet unforeseen emergencies."[26] Isn't that what it's all about?

Most older people aren't worried about dying so much as they're worried about losing their independence and their minds. Being physically active is the single best way to prevent those losses. Of particular benefit to older people is the potential for physical activity in a group setting to relieve the social isolation that is such a common problem in this population.

What Exercise is Best? Aerobic? Strength?

In general, the best exercise is one that you'll like enough to do regularly. For both younger and older people, a combination of aerobic and strength, or resistance, training is best. There are some other factors, though, that you may want to consider.

Aerobic Activity

Overall, aerobic exercise has the best mood-elevating effects for most people, particularly if the activity is done outdoors.[27, 28] Perhaps as a consequence, there seems to be greater adherence to outdoor exercise regimens compared with indoor ones.[29] If you enjoy walking but have knee pain due to osteoarthritis, consider walking more frequently but for shorter periods of time. You'll have less discomfort that way.[30]

Strength (Resistance) Training

Strength training, either with free weights or machines, helps protect against the loss of muscle mass and strength that is otherwise inevitable with growing older.[31] The importance of this training isn't to help you "bulk up" your muscles but to make it easier to lift a bag of groceries or get up out of a chair—that is, to live a vigorous, comfortable, independent life. Speaking of bulking up, if you most definitely do *not* want bulkier muscles, then lift lighter weights and do more repetitions. You're also less likely to experience strains and injuries that way.

Jae—I was surprised to discover that I love weight lifting. I had absolutely no idea what I was doing when I started out, but I enjoyed it and learned how to do it safely. I feel so damn powerful after lifting weights—like I can take on the world! As a single woman who's alone much of the time, I love feeling like I can protect myself better. I love the sense of independence when I can move apartments by myself because I can lift everything. I also love that the progress is tangible—I discovered I can usually add a little more weight every week, and I actually have visible muscles in my arms and back!

In summary, both forms of exercise are great, and a combination of aerobic and resistance exercise is ideal for both younger and older people.[32, 33]

Aquatic Exercise

Consider swimming or pool walking if you have muscle or joint pain. The load on joints and muscles is reduced by half or even more compared with land-based exercise.[34] Because of this, water exercise may be more comfortable and allow you to have greater range of motion and function.[35]

Use Motivators

Find a Buddy

Exercising with another person may be more fun for you and will also make you more accountable.

Jae—In Chapter 1, I mentioned how I began my exercise journey with my friend, Sarah, and how helpful it was for me to have that support and accountability. In the next chapter, I'll tell you specifically about how, with her encouragement, I got myself to a gym. I was able to share all of my insecurities, fears, and successes with Sarah; and she could do the same with me. I knew that if I were to give up, I would also be abandoning my friend. We were a team.

Make a Music Playlist

Janice—I have one playlist for when I use my hand weights or do floor exercises and another faster playlist for when I'm out walking to keep me from slowing down too much. I just hope no one ever sees me singing and bopping along when "Uptown Funk" comes on.

On the other hand, you may want to use your exercise as a time to think, reflect, and have some quiet time, in which case music may be distracting and annoying. Whatever works for you is the way to go.

Get Tech Support

An activity tracker such as a Fitbit or Apple Watch may be useful for you with regard to giving you feedback and also providing motivation to continue, and even increase, physical activity.[36]

Jae—I find using my Apple Watch motivating. I am a goal-oriented person, and I like using the app to help me set a goal each day for number of steps or calories burned. It also gives me a more accurate picture of my activity level. I also like that I can friend people in the app, which allows me to receive or give encouragement to other people. If you like, it can be a friendly competition with winning results no matter where you place!

Don't Let Exercise Be Another Source of Shame

We've established that exercise helps with weight, mood, and physical and mental health. Your body and your brain will thank you for being physically fit. Sounds good, right? But maybe you already knew all this, and you're wondering what good it does to *know* it if you're not actually going to *do* it? What if you don't exercise now because it just sounds too unpleasant or you are embarrassed by your body? We get that. Perhaps you are uncomfortable exercising in public, or you may not have the stamina to work out at home. But try. Go up some stairs today. Park a little farther away from the store. Learn how to use free weights, and buy some that are just heavy enough to use properly. Also, check out different types of exercise and see if any of them appeal to you.

Jae—I didn't even start to exercise until I had lost eighty pounds. So many people do not understand what it's like to feel trapped in a state of body shame. They've said to me, "Just eat less and move more." The equation is not that simple! It's physical, mental, and emotional. I needed to find my own way. I can't live without exercise now, but it didn't start out that way at all!

Janice—I'm not athletic. I'm not graceful. I never was. My body may not be beautiful, but I appreciate it all the same. I appreciate moving my body in ways that allow me to more fully participate in the world. And I can't tell you how much I appreciate being able to walk faster and further at age sixty-eight than I could at age fifty-eight.

Please don't say simply that you hate exercise and won't do it. Whatever you weigh, asking your body to move more is showing it kindness, respect, and appreciation. The physical and psychological effects are profound. It can enhance your family and social relationships. It prevents disease, it's free (or at least it can be), and it doesn't cause allergic reactions. What a prescription! The best way to stop being angry with your body is to incorporate physical activity into your life. In the next chapter, we'll take you through the steps of doing just that.

CHAPTER 19

Physical Exercise, Part 2—Your Action Plan

> "Exercise" doesn't have to be
> synonymous with "I hate this."

Everyone knows that exercise is good for their health. So why don't they do it regularly? The excuses are many: "I'm not athletic;" "I don't have time;" "I tried it once and didn't like it;" etc. It's a long list. You may have come up with some pretty terrific excuses yourself. But time's up. We're here to help you discover how to become physically active in a way that allows you to stick with it and that will not be another source of perceived failure and shame.

Do Something Achievable

Strive for your Personal Best. What's that? *Personal Best*, or *Personal Record* (PR), is a sports terms that refers to a person's best performance. We think it's a wonderful concept because you make the rules for yourself, and the results are tangible. Are you able to walk up five steps? Okay, then, that's your Personal Best. Now you can strive for six. The actual goal is much less important than feeling successful and motivated enough to keep trying.

Jae—*When I took up running, it wasn't about winning. However, I did strive to set new PRs—running just a little longer or a second faster than the time before. My PRs kept me motivated because I was competing against myself and nobody else. I love the feedback of seeing my improvement, which means that my efforts are paying off. I'll never be able to run a six-minute mile, but I sure as heck can try to run for ten seconds longer than the last time.*

Janice—*It's just fine with me that someone else can run up twenty flights of stairs and lift small cars. Good for them—but it has nothing to do with me. I just want to do better for* me. *Having said that, I really do try to push myself to hike a little farther, walk up a hill a little faster, or do a few more reps with my hand weights. And after I achieve that, I feel a great sense of satisfaction.*

Do Something You Like, At Least Sort Of

Jae loves running and weight lifting; Janice loves hiking and gardening. We both love to be outside. But this is about *you*. Find an activity you'll like enough to do regularly. Do you feel intimidated by the idea of going to a gym and seeing all those skinny, fit people who seem to look at you judgmentally? Fine—you don't have to go to a gym. Save your money, and go for a walk. Even in winter—perhaps *especially* in winter, we still recommend outdoor activity as long as it's not icy. As we talked about earlier, outdoor exercise tends to improve most people's mood even more than indoor exercise. Having said that, if you're more likely to stick with a routine of walking through a shopping mall, then that's the right activity for you. And if "having" to go for a walk feels like a forced march, then dance or do yoga or plant a bush. "Exercise" doesn't have to be synonymous with "I hate this." Just get moving!

Jae—A key to being successful is discovering what makes you tick. I am competitive with myself, so I enjoy striving to be stronger and faster in that spirit. Maybe you don't want to make this a competition, even with yourself. That's fine. We all got to where we are for different reasons and in different ways. Whether it's with exercise or weight loss, each one of us will set different goals and take different paths. As long as you don't give up and keep playing the long-term game, good things will happen. The relationship among food, your body, your mind, and your spirit will improve. You will feel more confident and powerful. I'm proof of that.

Janice—I cannot tell you how much money I wasted on gym memberships in the past, only to rediscover each time that I enjoyed going to the gym about as much as I enjoy going to the dentist. I used all my creative abilities to find excuses to stay home. It was the perfect setup for failure. But I love hiking with my dog and doing heavy garden work. Just because it's fun doesn't mean it isn't effective!

Speaking of fun, though, I now find myself back at a gym, thanks to Zumba Pete. For an hour, I'm moving and gasping to upbeat music and the most enthusiastic and least judgmental instructor in the world. Pete is a retired Broadway dancer. The people in his class do not have his resumé; we are of varied ages, sizes, and fitness levels. And we don't care about what anyone else is doing in the class. When Pete jumps, Janice marches. When Pete leaps, Janice—well, doesn't leap; I just do my best. And that's the point.

Make a Commitment

You can easily eat a bowl of ice cream every night without needing to make a commitment to do so. Exercise is different. If you ask yourself if you feel like exercising today, you may find yourself having a "good" reason to say no 90 percent of the time. So don't ask that question. We talked about habits in Chapter 13 and how connecting two behaviors helps you to develop new habits. It needs to be like that with exercise. You get up in the morning and go for a brisk walk before you shower. Or you stop at the gym on your way home from work. Or you get home, change your clothes, and do some work with weights. Or you join a hiking club. You get the idea.

Make a firm commitment and keep it: commit to going for a brisk walk for twenty minutes four days a week, or going to a dance class or to the swimming pool twice a week, or working with a personal trainer once a week. The choice is yours.

Janice—Here's how it works for me: I used to come home from work, change into comfortable clothes, and then make dinner and do whatever else I needed or wanted to do for the evening. Now, I come home, change into comfortable clothes and then, before, I do anything else, turn on music or the television and do exercises with my five-pound weights. I also do core and balance exercises and stretches. The whole thing takes twenty minutes. For me, having this become a nearly daily routine works better than doing a longer session less often. That's because it has developed into an automatic habit by now—I put on comfortable clothes and pick up the weights. If I'm feeling really unmotivated, I tell myself that I only have to do my exercises for ten minutes. When those ten minutes are up, though, I almost always want to keep going.

Jae—Doing what you enjoy makes it so much easier to develop a habit, and making a new habit helps you enjoy what you're doing. At first, I hated running. I tried an elliptical for twenty minutes and didn't come back for months! But once I tried it again and made it a habit, I started to love running. I never would have thought this was possible. The point is, find something you think you might possibly like, make it a habit, and see if you grow to like it enough to keep doing it.

Give Yourself Credit

When you come back home from your walk or when you put down your weights, congratulate yourself. Thank your body for doing a good job. And if you weren't physically active today, for whatever reason, don't beat yourself up. Make a plan to do something tomorrow.

What's the Best Way to Get Started? Just Start.

If you're just beginning, be sensible: don't get out of your chair for the first time and try to run five miles. Walk at a comfortable pace for five or ten minutes, and see how that feels. You can gradually increase your activity and walk a little farther and a little faster, but don't worry about it before you begin. Just start with a goal that seems reasonable to you in terms of how many minutes a day and how many days a week you intend to dedicate to it. If ten minutes twice a day is more enjoyable for you and easier to incorporate into your routine than twenty minutes once a day, that's the right choice. If you have medical problems, particularly risk factors for coronary artery disease, talk to your doctor before you start an exercise regimen.

Jae—When I first started running, I followed the C25K program. The first day of this program has you run for only sixty seconds, followed by walking for ninety seconds. There's no way I could have tried to run a mile at first, or even half a mile. I started small and worked my way up.

Maybe you can start by walking up a flight of stairs instead of taking the elevator. Or parking your car a little farther from the store. Or meeting a friend for a walk after dinner. Just start. Thank your body afterwards. Congratulate yourself. Repeat.

How Jae Got Started

Jae—*Walking into a gym when you're obese takes courage. I didn't start exercising until after I had already lost 80 pounds. I weighed 190 pounds when I first went to the gym. I had to wait until I was mentally, as well as physically, ready to start the process of introducing physical exercise into my daily routine. I hope that sharing my experience with you can help you see how it's possible to get started.*

First, I should explain why I even went to a gym in the first place. I had gotten to a point where I knew I wanted to incorporate exercise into the changes I was making in my life, but I still didn't feel confident enough to be "exposed" outside. The thought of that caused too much anxiety for me. I was a college sophomore, and my roommate encouraged me to go to the gym with her. Honestly, I would have found every excuse in the book to not go if it wasn't for this one invitation.

The first step of gym intimidation was the dressing room. All the people there looked so confident that they didn't even seem to care about who saw their bodies. That sure wasn't me! I had already eliminated this first hurdle, though, by changing in my dorm room ahead of time.

Then it was time to actually work out. My roommate said we'd do just twenty minutes on the elliptical to get our heart rates up and our legs warm. Easy for her to say—she looked like she belonged there. In order to be as invisible as possible, she and I went to the treadmills that were the furthest away from other people. Even so, it was very hard for me. I felt like I was being judged by everyone else in the room for being the "fat one" who would give up after two minutes. They probably thought

I was going to just huff and puff for those two minutes and then reward myself with a pint of Ben & Jerry's Half Baked ice cream on the way home. I thought they might be right.

Honestly, no one could be more surprised than I was that I lasted the whole twenty minutes. Don't get me wrong—my legs hurt like hell, and I felt like I'd completely run out of oxygen—but I also felt something new. I was proud of myself, and I felt like I had actually accomplished something significant. This definitely made me realize that doing physical exercise was possible, that I could actually keep going with this.

It wasn't that easy, though. I did not step foot in that gym for another two months after the first day. Things got in the way; life was too crazy. Honestly, I also have to admit that it was just so hard to even think about going to the gym again. But I still wanted to give myself credit for having had the courage to enter that gym, occupy the space there, and survive. I didn't want to let anybody's real or imagined judgment keep me from moving.

A month and a half after that first trip, I found the "C25K" or "Couch to 5K" Program on Reddit's /r/C25K forum. For some reason, I thought to myself, "Hell, I did twenty minutes on the elliptical and didn't die. I think I can at least try this, too."

I loved how little commitment was involved. Actually, that was my favorite part. Sarah, a friend from a club I was in at Penn, wanted to try it as well, which perfectly set us up as each other's accountability partner. In order to keep each other honest, we both signed up for a 5K race ten weeks out from our start date. We scheduled training runs in our calendars as though they were meetings so we couldn't make any excuses. I thrived with structure, and I was also motivated to show up because I knew how guilty I would feel if I stood Sarah up. We even went so far as to send each other photos of our feet on the treadmill if our schedules did not align! Our system really worked and was an important reason we were so successful together. By the time we finished training and ran the 5K race, we felt like we could do anything. I haven't stopped running since. Here's what I recommend for you, based on my experiences:

Listen to yourself. For me, exercising regularly was the same as losing weight: I needed to find my own way. You'll find your own way, too. As we talked about earlier in this chapter, find something that you like to do and that keeps you engaged and motivated. If running is not the best choice for you because it doesn't feel good for your body or is too damn boring, why run if you hate it? You're likely to not stick with it, and then you'll feel discouraged. Instead, try walking, biking, Zumba, swimming . . . the possibilities are endless.

I wish I could have convinced college sophomore Jae not to feel so much trepidation about going to the gym in the first place. There is nothing to be ashamed of when you step foot in the gym—you are there, and you're there for yourself. Yes, there may be an element of judgment of "fat people" at the gym, and it's hard to escape because of the bias in our society (which we're going to talk about in Chapter 25). Know that the people who are doing the judging are the ones who should be ashamed. Their judgment betrays their own insecurity, pettiness, and cruelty—but you don't have to give them the power to make you feel bad about yourself. You deserve to be in that gym just as much as anyone else. It took me a while to learn to change the negative energy I felt into motivation and dedication to my goal. I didn't even know it at the time, because it didn't seem achievable, but my goal simply became to stop hating my body. I achieved that goal. And I hope you can, too.

STEP EIGHT:

Learn Our Secrets, and Create Your Own

CHAPTER 20

Going Out to Eat with Janice & Jae

Whenever I allow myself to ask whether it's okay to eat something that I've decided ahead of time that I'm better off avoiding . . . I have found that I can always find a reason to answer, "Sure you can."

Have you ever entertained these thoughts when eating out?

- Here's that heavenly basket of warm, free bread. I can't just ignore it!
- Everyone is ordering dessert; I may as well, too. I don't want to stand out.
- Everything on this buffet looks so amazing—and I should get my money's worth.
- No one else at the table wants the rest of the wine; it's a shame to let it go to waste.

Food is so much more than fuel for the body. Eating is also a social activity, enhancing connections, pleasure, and relaxation. But eating out is full of traps that can sabotage your best intentions to become slimmer and healthier. We share your pain. Let's get through this together so you can enjoy yourself whenever you go out instead of suffering any self-recrimination afterward.

Strategies Before You Even Leave Your House or Workplace

First and foremost, don't let yourself be ambushed. Before you go to a restaurant, plan ahead. Here's what we mean:

- If you know where you are going, look at the menu beforehand. Take the time to read it and consider your options. Many restaurants have detailed nutritional information available— use this to your advantage. Consider ahead of time what you'd like to order while you're not under any pressure, instead of making the decision when you're ravenously hungry and your friends are waiting for you to order.
- You may want to call the restaurant to see if they can accommodate substitutions (such as green vegetables for fries). The more planning you do in advance, the more mindful you'll be when you order and the less disappointed you'll feel after you eat.

Janice—*I love the idea of looking at a restaurant menu beforehand. For me, it becomes part of enjoying the restaurant experience, and, most of all, it gives me time to calmly make healthy choices. But I have to stick to my guns. I make sure I don't change my mind once I'm at the restaurant. I order the food that I planned for, enjoy every bit of what I eat, and congratulate myself afterward for handling the situation like a grown-up.*

Jae—*I also love planning ahead when I eat out because it helps me reduce anxiety around making good food choices, as well as the possible social anxiety I sometimes still feel about eating with other people. Additionally, when I find myself just staring at the menu for three minutes before making a choice, I find that I miss items or feel too rushed to make an informed decision, which can lead to picking an item because it's something I've liked before, rather than the right pick. When I go into these situations with a plan already set out, then I don't have to think about anything. No anxiety. I can eat what I planned, feel confident in my decision, and focus on being present and engaged with my company. This makes the experience so much more enjoyable.*

Advocate for Yourself

If you haven't had time to call ahead, then once you get to the restaurant, advocate for yourself and your food choices by ordering what *you* want without worrying that other people will think you're "asking for too much." Just check with your waiter—the restaurant will let you know if they cannot accommodate you. What if your friends make comments about you being "difficult" or making too many requests? If you are comfortable with saying so, let them know those comments make you feel like they are undermining your decision to be healthier and more cognizant of what you eat. Or simply shrug and smile. Or ignore the comments altogether. You have every right to take care of yourself.

Jae—*During this process of creating new habits and trying out new strategies, you're going to be putting in a lot of time to figure out what works for you. To help keep track of it all, use your cell phone. Make a note or memo in your phone that's dedicated purely to restaurants. When you find a dish you like, write it down. Include nutrition information if you're tracking calories, any substitutions you made, etc. That way, everything is saved in an easily accessible log. It doesn't have to be pretty—it just needs to work for you. When you're in a new place, if you have a list of personally "preapproved" meals, you can use it as a reference to find the most similar item on the menu.*

Stimulus Control When There Are Overwhelming Stimuli

Janice—My Evil Twin loves going out to eat—and she very much wants to express her opinions when I'm looking at a menu. If my eyes land on the "crispy" (code word for "breaded and fried") chicken wings, and if I allow my eyes to linger on that item for even a few seconds to give my brain time to consider ordering them, my Evil Twin will seize the opportunity and tell me, "Go ahead; you're here to have fun. Tomorrow, you can have lettuce for dinner. What's the point of going out if you can't eat what you want?"

When I'm staring at the fried chicken wings option, that question about why I should not order what I want seems completely reasonable. But if I think clearly about it beforehand, I can answer the question differently:

- *The point of going out to eat with other people is to connect socially over a meal.*
- *I can still enjoy any meal without derailing my intention of eating in a healthy way.*
- *More than that, "eating what I want" means something different to me now. What I want is to eat in a way that takes care of my physical and emotional health.*

Whenever I allow myself to ask whether it's okay to eat something that I've decided ahead of time that I'm better off avoiding (say, fries or chocolate cake), I have found that I can always find a reason to answer, "Sure you can." So, I just don't go there. I go into the restaurant telling myself that I will not eat fries or cake today. It doesn't mean I'm no longer allowed to eat fries or cake forever; it simply means I've made a choice today, and I'm going to commit to it. This makes my life much easier and less stressful. What's more, it gives me the chance to focus on spending time with my friends, the more important reason for me to eat out in the first place.

Please don't confuse this strategy with a pity-party. We are not suggesting that you can never eat the fried wings. Rather, we're suggesting that you may not want to eat them *today*. The future is up to you. We can assure you, though, that as you reap the rewards of healthier eating habits, you'll be less and less likely to desire the unhealthy items on the menu.

Jae's Restaurant Action Plan

What if you don't know where you're going ahead of time? Jae has her own approach to navigating new menus and restaurants.

Jae—I'm like Janice—one of the things I know about myself is that if the possibility is there to eat a certain food, I'm really, really good at coming up with convincing arguments for all the reasons why I should allow myself to eat it. So, I have had to come up with ways to avoid falling into traps when I go out to eat. One thing I do is focus on my guidelines for restaurants. Janice touched on it before when she talked about the chicken wings, but I take an extra step.

When I get a menu at a restaurant, the first thing I do is mentally block out desserts, unless there's fresh fruit. I can have deserts, but I have them on my own terms.

Next, I block out any pasta dishes, treating them as if they do not exist. Sure, there may be a whole page dedicated to all the wonderful variations of penne and spaghetti, but they're not for me. Like Janice mentioned, I'm not saying you can never, ever have pasta in your life; what matters here is your choice in the moment. I ignore pasta for a few reasons: one, restaurants rarely serve just one reasonable serving of pasta; second, most pasta is prepared with a lot of oil and/or butter. If I'm going to eat pasta, I save it for when I'm in charge in the kitchen, when I know exactly what and how much of everything is going into my pasta dish.

Next is fried foods. Hell, yeah, they're freaking amazing. That's why they're on nearly every restaurant menu! But are they going to help me reach my goals? No. Do I need them right now at this very instant? No. So they're out.

Next I look at anything high in starches, like potatoes. I know that if I eat a starch-heavy meal, I won't feel great, and I'll get hungry again fairly quickly. So there go all the potato-heavy dishes.

Lastly, I ignore anything that's heavily cheese-based. Cheese isn't bad, but a dish made with lots of cheese and cream is not going to help me reach or sustain my goals. At the end, I have a good list of dishes to pick from.

Other rules I make for myself include:

- *I eat all sandwiches with no bun. Instead of ordering the sandwich as-is and leaving the bun uneaten, I ask the waiter to serve it without the bun because I know myself—if it's there, I'm going to eat it. I make sure the choice isn't even on the table.*
- *I look for meals that are high in protein.*
- *My side order is always salad or vegetables.*
- *It's okay to make up a meal from appetizers and sides.*
- *I always drink water, seltzer water, unsweetened tea, or coffee.*

What does this look like in practice? Here is a sample menu from a "Generic American Restaurant" to practice on.

Generic American Restaurant	
Starters	**Sides**
Onion Rings	Roasted Vegetables
Spinach Artichoke Dip	French Fries
Chips and Salsa	Mashed Potatoes
Baked Chicken Wings	Grilled Corn on the Cob
Mozzarella Sticks	Sautéed Mushrooms
Soup and Salads	**Beverages**
Loaded Chili with Potato	Soda
Tomato Basil Soup	Iced Tea (Sweetened)
Grilled Chicken Salad with Vinaigrette	Lemonade
Strawberry Walnut Salad	Coffee
Caesar Salad	Cappuccino
Mains	**Dessert**
Chicken Tenders	Milkshake (Chocolate/Vanilla/Strawberry)
Turkey Wrap	Sundae
Cheeseburger with Bacon and a Fried Egg	Carrot Cake
Grilled Chicken Sandwich	Skillet Brownie with Ice Cream
Spaghetti and Meatballs	Giant Cookie

First, no desserts! No to all of them. Even that warm gooey brownie. Actually, especially that warm gooey brownie. If fruit salad was on the menu, I might order that.

Second, no pasta dishes. Goodbye, spaghetti and meatballs.

Third, no fried foods. Farewell, onion rings, mozzarella sticks, chicken tenders, cheeseburger, and French fries. That one hurt a little bit.

Next, starch-heavy foods. That means chips and salsa, loaded chili with potato, mashed potatoes, and grilled corn on the cob.

Lastly, cheese-based foods. I already said no to mozzarella sticks, and I have to add the spinach artichoke dip because I know it's in a gloppy cream sauce.

Generic American Restaurant	
Starters	**Sides**
Onion Rings	Roasted Vegetables
Spinach Artichoke Dip	French Fries
Chips and Salsa	Mashed Potatoes
Baked Chicken Wings	Grilled Corn on the Cob
Mozzarella Sticks	Sautéed Mushrooms
Soup and Salads	**Beverages**
Loaded Chili with Potato	Soda
Tomato Basil Soup	Iced Tea (Sweetened)
Grilled Chicken Salad with Vinaigrette	Lemonade
Strawberry Walnut Salad	Coffee
Caesar Salad	Cappuccino
Mains	**Dessert**
Chicken Tenders	Milkshake (Chocolate/Vanilla/Strawberry)
Turkey Wrap	Sundae
Cheeseburger with Bacon and a Fried Egg	Carrot Cake
Grilled Chicken Sandwich	Skillet Brownie with Ice Cream
Spaghetti and Meatballs	Giant Cookie

Are you thinking that I've crossed out almost everything? In fact, I'm actually left with a great selection. Under starters, I'd be inclined to keep the baked *chicken wings on the table. The soups and salads section leaves me with tomato basil soup, grilled chicken salad, strawberry walnut salad, and Caesar salad. For a main course, I would choose between the turkey wrap and grilled chicken sandwich (without the bun). If there had been grilled fish or shrimp on the menu, I would have ordered that. Sides are roasted vegetables or sautéed mushrooms.*

My final order might be the grilled chicken sandwich without the bun, and a salad for the side. If I'm still hungry, I get a side of roasted veggies. I'm not at this restaurant to have the food experience of my life. If I were, then I'd be paying more than fifteen dollars for my meal. But this is just a regular restaurant, for a regular meal, for no special reason other than to spend time with friends. While there's still a part of me that wants the fried foods and desserts, I know that part of me doesn't have my best interests at heart.

Navigating a Buffet

Jae—You really need to have a strategy when you're at a buffet. I start with a plate of salad and/or vegetables. I eat all of that. Then I go back to the buffet to pick out the rest of what I'm going to eat, and I impose my just-one-plate rule. This means I don't go back to the buffet again and again and again. By having the first plate of veggies, I've started my meal in a positive mindset because I've already made a good choice. Furthermore, I've created more time to think about what I'm going to eat next, so I'm not overwhelmed by everything that's out there and not as hungry when I'm making those decisions.

On the Road with Jae

Jae—When I'm going on a road trip, I check my phone ahead of time for places along the way. Then I go to my handy list stored in my phone, look at what I'm going to order, and stick to my plan. What happens when I can't plan ahead? I always keep a "cheat sheet" of things I have ordered from popular restaurant chains. That means that whenever I have a surprise visit somewhere, I already know what I'm going to have. This way, I eliminate the stress of a spur-of-the-moment food decision that might be one I'll regret. If I'm traveling with other people and I'm not hungry, I just order something to drink or a coffee. I remind myself that just because other people are eating does not mean I have to mindlessly follow along.

Sometimes, the only choice is a gas station mini-mart. Here, I like to look for items that have protein (which is filling), that are easy to eat, and that are as unprocessed as possible. I look for things like almonds, yogurt, or cheese sticks. I like lite popcorn (not the super salty over buttery ones or white cheddar, as tempting as they are). I also look for fruit that's easy to eat in the car, like apples and bananas. When I'm in a fix, I'll choose a protein bar, preferably one with more protein and less sugar.

*When it comes to air travel, I never eat airline food, even for long-haul flights. Think back to the last time you were on a plane—was the airline food memorable (in a good way)? I'm going to guess not. **Just because they give you free food does not mean you have to eat it.** This applies to all aspects of your life and other free-food situations. If you're going to be spending the day traveling, take food with you. I like to pack carrots, apple slices, grapes, nuts, cheese sticks, hardboiled eggs, protein bars, or a combination of those. All of these will pass through airport security and are easy snacks that are more than enough to satisfy me. For something more substantial, I find something at a restaurant on the other side of security and bring it onto the plane with me.*

We hope Jae's strategy feels workable and helpful to you. This is a good time for a new list.

List #10: Travel Foods

You make a list of things to bring with you when you're going on a trip, right? How about including foods to take with you that will help keep your healthy intentions from being sabotaged?

Finally, remember that you're a work in progress, just as we are. You may find yourself in a restaurant when you're tired, anxious, worried, and stressed—and you're ordering a second martini. And a cheesesteak. And then, since you've "blown it," a hot fudge sundae. We hope it was all delicious and that, now, you want to move forward with healthier food choices and healthier stress management strategies. That's it. No guilt or shame. Move forward with your new life.

CHAPTER 21

Holidays, Parties, and Other Potential Catastrophes

> Don't treat the holiday as though
> it's a surprise party. Plan what
> you're going to eat ahead of time.

Holiday gatherings, parties, and vacations all have in common the abundance of delicious food. We think you should enjoy yourself and enjoy the food. However, if "enjoying yourself" means eating in a way that feels out of control, then that "enjoyment" will be awfully short-lived, especially if it derails your best intentions for feeling in charge of how and what you eat. It can be difficult, of course. Food isn't merely fuel—it's part of the fabric that makes up our families and cultures. We eat not just for sustenance, but for pleasure, for celebration of rituals and shared experiences, and for the joy of being with others. For some people, eating sensibly in social situations is easy; but for the rest of us, these occasions can be landmines of temptation and emotional eating, where the food outweighs the love and togetherness, leaving you with self-recrimination that's even harder to digest than all those calories.

Holidays—Ho, Ho, Ho

As wonderful as the holidays can be—family time, shared memories, beautiful traditions—they can also represent a special circle of hell. Buttons get pressed, old wounds resurface, and the emotional temperature can be just too damn hot. Adults become children again, and not in a good way. Don't despair, though—there's a lot you can do to keep the food and the negative emotions in control.

Janice & Jae's Holiday Survival Kit

Have you ever found yourself "somehow" eating until you realized you stopped being hungry an hour ago and you now feel mentally numb and physically ill? What kind of holiday was that? There's a simple way to prevent the misery: don't treat the holiday as though it's a surprise party. *Plan* what you're going to eat *ahead of time*. We're not saying that you should have nothing on your plate except string beans and a slice of dry turkey on Thanksgiving; that would be just plain sad. On the other hand, you may not want to eat a third helping of buttery sweet potatoes with marshmallows. Or, maybe that's exactly what you *want* to do. Go right ahead—it's your choice. The point is, we strongly recommend that you make a conscious decision about what you plan to eat beforehand. Go ahead and enjoy that second piece of pumpkin pie—if that is what you had planned to eat. Don't have it on the spur of the moment just because, you know, what the hell.

Reinforce Your Game Plan

Here are some specifics about planning ahead:

- If you're going to someone else's place for Thanksgiving, plan what you're going to eat before you even leave your house.

One helping of stuffing? One scoop of sweet potato casserole? One piece of pie or two? One glass of wine or three? It's your decision.

- Offer to bring some food. That way you have at least one item you can plan on that is reliable and that you know you will feel good about eating. Bring something healthy and delicious, such as roasted sweet potatoes or green vegetables that aren't slathered in gloppy sauce.

- Don't arrive hungry. Before you leave your house, have a healthy snack or small meal, like salad or vegetable soup.

- When you sit down, look around and further refine your plan. First, locate the vegetables—the healthy ones, like the vegetables you brought. Put a lot of them on your plate. Then some turkey, preferably without the skin. Then a little bit of everything else.

- As we'll discuss in detail in the next chapter, our strategy for **every single meal is to eat all the healthy vegetables first.** By doing this, we fill up on the healthiest, least calorie-dense foods so that we're no longer ravenously hungry when we dig into the rest. We can't emphasize enough how helpful this has been for us.

- Then it's time for dessert. Cousin Susan makes the best pumpkin pie in the world? It's Thanksgiving, so go ahead and have some—but only according to what you had planned ahead of time. You could plan to share a piece, or have one piece for yourself without the crust, or have two pieces with the crust and topped with extra whipped cream. It's your choice—as long as you plan what you eat in advance and then eat exactly that amount. Enjoy every single bite, and congratulate yourself for staying with your plan. Give yourself credit. By doing this, you can walk away from the table feeling positive about your food decisions and feeling proud of yourself.

Jae—*Every year at Christmastime, and only then, my aunt makes her famous chocolate walnut fudge. This fudge is bomb. It's truly special. So, you know what I do? I have a piece. I enjoy it. I eat it slowly. I savor it. I allow myself to be happy that I was able to experience it. I don't feel deprived, and I'm proud of myself for eating in a sane way.*

Janice—*That's how I feel about Passover seders. No, it's not the matzoh—I don't know a single soul who craves matzoh. It's those chocolate-covered coconut macaroons. Oh my. I used to end the festive meal in a far-from-festive food coma. Now, I plan ahead to have only one macaroon—and when I eat it, I'm in heaven. Then it's time to kiss everyone goodbye and head on home.*

You may be delighted to find that there's been a paradigm shift: **you're eating what you want to eat, but you've changed the meaning of what you want to eat.**

Next suggestion: **slow it down**. There's always too much to do before a holiday, which is a given. Figure out strategies to both minimize the stress and to deal with it in a self-caring way. Sleep is not a luxury, but rather a sanity saver. If making the sixth batch of Christmas cookies is going to hurl you over the edge of reason, five batches are enough. If you can't find the perfect gift, give an okay gift with a heartfelt card. If there are too many presents to wrap, get bags and tissue paper. You get the idea. Keep it jolly.

Stress Busters

Holiday preparations can put you over the top with regard to stress. Too much stress will take all the fun out of a holiday and wear down your emotions and your body. Here's a little recap from Chapters 15 and 18:

1. Bump up the exercise

Exercise just means getting your heart rate elevated (and not by getting into argument with your sister-in-law). It can be as simple as a ten-minute walk around the block—or several a day, if you can. Being outside in the daytime is an even more potent mood-elevator as the days get shorter.

2. Set aside downtime to reboot

Meditation, yoga, or even just closing your eyes and taking deep, slow breaths for three minutes can make a difference. You can also jot down three things that you're thankful for that morning—anything to help you keep your heart rate down and your jaw unclenched.

3. Expand the space between stimulus and response

Translation: when a toxic family member starts spewing the usual poison, you don't have to drink it this time. Pause before you respond, or don't respond at all. In fact, you can plan ahead of time how you want to deal with a difficult relative. Don't give that person the power to undermine your efforts, goals, and dignity. You deserve better than that.

4. Stick with your intentions

For whatever reasons, there will be "loved ones" and "friends" who seem determined to sabotage your efforts with what can feel like force-feeding. "Oh, come on," they say, insisting on spooning the third helping of stuffing onto your plate. "You can eat this." Well, yes, you can eat this, but shouldn't that be *your* decision?

Jae—Better yet, plan an exit strategy in the event that you feel over-whelmed. When I was at home during the holidays and felt the tension

196

building, my exit strategy was my dog. If I felt like I was on the verge of calling out a family member and knew the conversation would deteriorate from there, I would politely excuse myself and say that the dog needed to go outside. Nobody needed to know that our dog was really just walking laps in the backyard with me.

Halloween: A Special Circle of Hell for Us Candy Lovers

Here's a Halloween haiku:

Only six years old.
She hid her candy from me.
Found it. Sorry, Jo.

Janice—Yes, it's true. When my daughter Joanna was just six, I rummaged through her room to find the Halloween candy she had hidden from me. The scene that followed humiliates me to this day. Let's just say that I'm very, very lucky she has a forgiving and kind nature. But for all of us who have a "problem," shall we say, with sugary foods, Halloween is very tough. Which is why I'm offering you the following Halloween "recipe" to make after the last trick-or-treater has darkened your doorstep:

- Bring all the leftover candy into the kitchen.
- Unwrap each piece.
- Throw the candy in the garbage.
- Throw stuff over it—vinegar, mustard, whatever.
- Bag up the garbage.
- Take it outside.
- Pat yourself on the back.
- Smile. Go to bed.

Jae—*For me, the most effective way to avoid snacking on Halloween candy meant for trick-or-treaters is to buy only candy that I dislike. For example, I hate Twizzlers—so my candy bowl is filled with them. I also keep cut apples by the door so that if for some reason I feel tempted when the kids come to the door, I can take a piece of apple. This makes me feel so much better about my choices, and I go to bed feeling proud of myself.*

Two years ago, I was a champ. I made it through Halloween, and I was feeling good about sticking to my goals—until I fell victim to the after-Halloween candy sale. Seventy-five percent off candy? What a deal! I can never resist a good deal. I bought a bag of Reese's pumpkins and demolished them. They tasted amazing in the moment, but afterward, I felt awful. Last year, determined to avoid the temptation, I told myself a little lie: "All the candy is on sale because it's past the expiration date." Is it true? Who's to say? All I know is it worked for me, and I'm sticking with that story this year.

If you eat a piece of candy (or more), don't be discouraged. It's just one little blip in the big picture. Don't forget, one mistake does not mean you are a screw-up. All it means is you are human. Treat yourself with kindness, forgive yourself, and remember that November 1 is a new day. New habits take time. Give yourself a break.

We suggest that you make a list to fine-tune your own strategies for negotiating difficult social and emotional terrain during the holidays.

List #11: Strategies for Getting through Holidays

Since this time can be emotionally fraught, your journal can be really helpful. Before you "celebrate," write down some wonderful—and not-so-wonderful—things about previous holiday gatherings. What can you do differently this year, not just with regard to food, but also with regard to family dynamics? After the holiday is over, write your reflections. How was it this year? How did you take care of yourself emotionally, and how did your eating reflect that? What changes do you want to make in the future (and, no, you cannot switch families)?

Janice—*One last thing about holidays. My personal favorite food holiday is June 1. My mother's last meal was a cheeseburger. She was eighty-five years old, and she drove to a restaurant to have lunch with her friends, where she told them, "I know I shouldn't, but I'm going to have a cheeseburger." And so every year, on June 1, the anniversary of her death, I have a cheeseburger. If I'm in the mood, I even have the fries, too. And while I'm eating that plate of delicious fat and flesh, I thank her for not having had tofu for her last meal. I really, really enjoy that cheeseburger, and it's the last one I eat—until next June 1.*

Enjoy the Party

Parties are much the same as holidays—maximize your opportunities to enjoy yourself by doing your homework ahead of time. **Plan** what you're going to eat before you even get to the party. One burger? One handful of chips? A taste of potato salad? A beer or three glasses of wine? Again, it's your decision. You certainly don't want to wander into that mindset of deprivation, but we do recommend that you don't plan on having eight beers or glasses of wine—you may not be able to think clearly enough to keep your resolve.

Offer to bring vegetables, such as carrot, celery, or jicama sticks; bell pepper slices; broccoli pieces; etc., and a healthy dip, such as hummus or guacamole (there's no law that says you're only allowed to eat guacamole with chips!). Do you think a party is a total waste of time without chicken wings? Then enjoy the wings! But plan how many you're going to eat ahead of time, and stick to it. And that will be much easier to accomplish if you fill up on the vegetables first.

Jae—*Here's one of my strategies: at large social gatherings, there is typically a lot of food that tends to be on display. I use this to my advantage. Remember how we talked about buying time and using the time to reframe food choices? I take the time to survey and make a plan right in that moment by looking at every single food item before deciding what to eat. Then I take a plate and fill it first with vegetables and other healthy foods. After I've eaten and am already partially full, I go back with a smaller plate and take the other foods I have decided to eat.*

Take a Vacation, But Not from Your Best Intentions

Being on vacation is an opportunity for leisure, fun, and new experiences. A vacation may also be an opportunity for healthy moving and eating. How nice to come back from a break and feel rested and refreshed instead of wondering how it was possible to have eaten that much crap and gained that much weight in so short a time.

Sometimes you don't have a choice. When you're in Paris, all they may serve for breakfast is a croissant and coffee. Well, you'll just have to take one for the team and enjoy that flaky croissant. But lots of times, you will have choices. Consider these as you plan your trip:

- Stay at a place where there's a refrigerator and microwave so you can prepare your own food. You can have oatmeal or eggs for breakfast and keep fruit and yogurt in the fridge. If you have nothing more than a bed in your hotel room, you can still keep nuts and seeds for snacks.
- Think of how you can incorporate physical activity into your vacation. Physical fatigue is the most wonderful antidote to

mental fatigue. Maybe you'd like to try a day hike, or a walking tour instead of a bus tour of a city.

- Part of the fun of vacation is the food, especially new and local foods. Be adventurous, and enjoy yourself. But also use your tools and strategies to do so intelligently.
- Before you leave on your trip, plan where you'll eat on the way to your destination. While you're on the road, use your smartphone to help you find a suitable place to eat or bring food along with you. And be sure to bring healthy snacks for the car or plane—carrot sticks, nuts, apple slices, etc. Have a great trip!

CHAPTER 22

Jae & Janice's Secrets

> If there is a plate of cookies in front of us,
> we both feel "hungry" for those cookies until
> the plate is empty. Our intuition simply isn't
> trustworthy in the world of processed foods.

Secrets? There aren't any. Really. No "miracle cure," no sit-on-your-butt-and-eat-all-the-crap-you-want-and-lose-weight diet. We're simply going to tell you what worked, and continues to work, *for us*. It took each of us a while to take all the confusing and contradictory advice that's out there and distill it into something that's been useful for several years, and we hope it's beneficial for you, too. Use what helps you to eat in a physically and emotionally healthy way, and ignore or modify what doesn't.

Secret #1: We Don't Ambush Ourselves

If you behave in a way that causes you regret later, and if you repeat that behavior a hundred times, then why would you think that the hundred and first time is going to be different? Why put yourself in that position again?

Impulsive Eating Is Dangerous—For Us

In Chapter 11, we talked about how *increasing* the space between stimulus and response is a powerful tool for seizing control over what you eat (as well as affecting how you interact with people, how you think, and how you view the world). *Shortening* that space, on the other hand, is what leads to impulsive, mindless eating and a sense of things spiraling out of control.

Janice—I cannot allow myself to eat impulsively. On most days, I plan in the morning so I know what prep I need to do and what I'll be eating for the rest of the day, as well as what the total number of calories will be. No mindless random grabbing at food, and no impetuous decisions. Isn't this system boring, you wonder? No, it isn't; I like the process of planning how I'm going to take good care of myself. Doesn't this strategy take out all the spontaneity associated with eating? Yes, it does, but that's the whole point, for me. I make a plan, carry it out, enjoy my food thoroughly and without any guilt, and pat myself on the back for sticking to the plan. Who knows, I might not have to be this rigid forever. But honestly, it doesn't feel like rigidity to me; it feels like calming, comforting structure. Most of all, I know that I won't have to be at war with my body for the rest of my life, and that's good enough for me.

For many people, and certainly for us, the best way to prevent unhealthy impulsive eating is to avoid having those foods available in the first place—*and* to have nutritious foods available and convenient, as we discussed in Chapter 9.

Moderation Doesn't Work—For Us

That sounds counterintuitive, doesn't it? The conventional "wisdom" is that you can eat anything you want, but in moderation. That's fine—for some people. If you're like us, though, eating a small amount of some unhealthy, delicious food isn't satisfying at all—you just crave a much larger amount. For us, it's better to just avoid those foods altogether—except, perhaps, on special occasions that we've designated as special ahead of time.

Jae—There are certain foods that are just not allowed in my house. Ever. For example, I know that if I have a sleeve of Oreos or a bag of tortilla chips at home, I will eat every single cookie or chip in one sitting. Same thing with a chocolate bar or peanut butter. But here's the point I want to make: since I know this about myself, I have devised strategies so I don't put myself in a situation where this becomes an issue. Not even little prepackaged single servings are allowed (because, honestly, I don't care one bit if it's individually packaged and there's nothing stopping me from going back to the box and grabbing another one). This doesn't mean I will not allow myself to eat cookies, tortilla chips, chocolate, or peanut butter ever again; I just do not allow these foods in my house where they are easily accessible.

If I want any of these things, it has to be because 1) someone has offered it to me; 2) it is served in a restaurant; or 3) I have utilized my "active plan" to get it. What's my active plan? As mentioned in Chapter 9, I select a convenience store approximately two miles away from my house, even if there's one just three blocks away, and walk there to get what I want. This makes getting that food item a big commitment and effort, and if I decide to follow through, it helps me to get some exercise. When I get to the store, I allow myself to buy only a single-serving size—I'm not going down the bulk candy aisle!

I used to see a nutritionist to help me work on my eating habits once I started maintaining my weight. At the time, I was a Residence Advisor in a dorm that had a fresh-baked cookie night every Wednesday, and my supervisor encouraged me to attend so I could bond with my residents. It was literally hell for me. We're talking four-hundred-plus cookies spread out in a room—and I was supposed to just stand there and watch other people eat them! My nutritionist told me, "Just let yourself have one." Here's the problem: I know I'm not going to have just one; I'm going to have one plus one plus one, to the point where I have cookie amnesia. I soon learned that if I was going to be successful, I had to be all or nothing. The negative feeling of watching everyone eat cookies was a whole lot less negative than hating myself for eating one damn cookie after another.

Janice—In order to cut down on eating sugary processed foods, I had to stop completely. When I tried to cut down, I was overwhelmed with "needing" more. I learned that a gradual decrease was impossible—for me. Remember that there's not just one right way to do this. You'll find your own way. Just be sure that it feels like a positive change for yourself and not like permanent deprivation.

Intuitive Eating Doesn't Work—For Us

Intuitive eating refers to paying attention to your body's inner hunger cues, rather than to external food cues. That sounds sensible, doesn't it? The problem is, while it may be sensible, it may not be achievable. Even today, neither of us is able to distinguish between those two types of cues when we're faced with delicious, sweet, fatty, salty foods. If there is a plate of cookies in front of us, we both feel "hungry" for those cookies until the plate is empty. Our intuition simply isn't trustworthy in the world of processed foods.

Jae—Even now that I've lost all that weight, I still can't interpret hunger cues. A nutritionist tried to teach me about intuitive eating, where you pay attention to your body's hunger signals and where you are on the "hunger-fullness scale." On one end, number one, is "starving," and on the other, ten, is "so full that you are going to puke." You're supposed to stay in the four to seven range. Unfortunately, for me, I can't find this middle ground. I only know when I'm so hungry that I feel light-headed and ready to pass out, and then there is the feeling of I-think-I'm-going-to-burst. Instead of being able to intuit when I am comfortably satisfied in order to stop, my brain is only able to register the moment of "there is food on this plate, and it's not gone yet, so more is going to go in my mouth." This was one of the reasons I got to 270 pounds. I could ignore literally every physical cue that my body was giving me to stop. This continues to be a problem for me, and it's something I have to actively work against every single day, every single time I eat.

Secret #2: We Know What Foods Work for Us—And When

Let's say you decide that a good general snack idea would be celery with some peanut butter on it. We agree—there are healthy nutrients and filling fiber in the celery, plus some protein and deliciousness in the peanut butter. But if you really hate celery and can only force it down your throat by covering it with half a jar of peanut butter, or if you feel unable to resist having a large mouthful of peanut butter every single time you open the pantry door to get something else, then celery with peanut butter may *not* be a good snack idea—for *you*.

In that spirit, we'll now share with you some of the food-related secrets to our success in the hope that they'll inspire you to discover your own.

We Eat Our Vegetables

We talked about vegetables in detail in the Chapter 17, and we've got to say it again: we are convinced that vegetables are the only solution to the riddle of how to eat enough food to be satisfied while consuming the right number of calories to lose weight in a healthy way.

Janice—When it comes to vegetables, my "secret" is that when I sit down to eat a meal, I eat all the vegetables first before I eat anything else. This does two things:

1. I fill up on the healthiest, least calorie-dense foods first.
2. I buy time between feeling like I could eat everything that's on the table, including the table itself, and feeling like a rational human being who can make healthy choices and eat in a sane, intentional way. It takes about twenty minutes for the brain to register that the stomach is getting full, so this extra time makes all the difference.

I try to eat some kind of vegetable before every meal. Ideally, I eat a vegetable or a salad with water or vegetable soup twenty minutes before sitting down to have lunch or dinner. Even if I don't feel like I'm "in the mood" for, say, a salad, if I am really hungry, once I start eating the salad, it starts to feel awfully satisfying after all, and then I'm filled up on it.

Jae—These are strategies I also use. Once I've eaten a lot of veggies, I start to feel full. The time that I've bought myself helps my brain to catch up. Since I'm halfway there, it's much easier to limit the portions of the less healthy, more calorie-dense foods that might be part of the meal.

In Chapter 9, I talked about keeping foods in their serving dishes and on the counter (instead of on the table), or even in the fridge in leftover containers. Not only does that keep me from taking second helpings mindlessly, it also gives me time to reflect on which choice I really want to make. Another reason this is successful is because once I've made a good food choice, it's much more compelling to keep making healthy choices and "continue the streak."

When I get home from the grocery store, I cut all of my veggies and fruit and put them away in plastic containers, instead of putting them *away whole. Even though this means they may not last quite as long, it works for me because I know I'm more likely to cook with them and add them to my meals once they are cut because of the convenience factor—the less prep time with my busy schedule, the better. To add interest and nutrition, I try to have as many colors of the rainbow present on my plate.*

Janice—I love pasta, and eating just a small portion of it doesn't work for me one bit. So what I do now is "spiralize" a big batch of zucchini or cook a spaghetti squash and toss in just a little cooked whole-wheat pasta. Next, I pile on a mound of vegetables that I've roasted in olive oil (which becomes the pasta sauce). Finally, I add my protein—beans, shrimp, or whatever—and it's fantastic!

Speaking of veggies, fruits and vegetables are the only foods I allow myself to eat while I'm standing up. That applies to when I'm preparing a meal, but also to when I'm clearing a meal. I can't even imagine how many calories I have mindlessly ingested from my family's plates while clearing their dishes from the table to the sink.

I also allow myself to eat all the fruit I want without counting calories because I know fruit is healthy, and the fiber in it makes it filling.

Breakfast. Hmm.

Some studies[1, 2] show that eating a healthy breakfast is a good idea if you want to lose weight in a healthy way. However, we have to admit that neither of us ate breakfast while we were losing weight. We both found that we seemed hungrier for the rest of the day whenever we ate breakfast. Again—do whatever works for you.

Janice—I do think that some of the new studies are compelling enough to make me rethink my strategy. One study showed that insulin seems to function more efficiently earlier in the day,[3] which means that eating a meal in the morning might result in less fat deposit than an identical meal eaten in the evening. Another study[4] supported that finding by showing that in two groups of women who were given identical foods and calories, those who ate most of their calories at breakfast lost two and a half times as much as those who ate most of the calories at dinner. The first group also had lower triglyceride and glucose levels and less abdominal fat. To top it all off, the breakfast people experienced less hunger throughout the day. The study author commented, "We observed that the time of the meal is more important than what you eat and how much you eat—it's more important than anything else in regulating metabolism." Yet another recent study[5] showed that skipping breakfast is associated with more low-grade inflammation and impaired glucose metabolism. Plus, most studies done with children recommend breakfast for this age group.[6, 7]

Upon reflection, I decided to eat a couple of tablespoons of yogurt with nuts and berries every morning. Even though I had already successfully lost weight and maintained the weight loss without breakfast, the health benefits seem good enough for me to want to start my day with a little protein, fiber, and vitamin-rich foods. I'm still waiting for a study to come along that recommends hot fudge sundaes as a healthy breakfast option . . .

However, skipping lunch is, for most people and certainly for me, a terrible idea. I've had patients tell me that sometimes, on busy days, they just "forget to eat" and "make up for it later." Forget to eat? Okay, I guess some people really are like that. But in this case, two things are likely to happen: one, when you get around to "remembering," you're so hungry that you literally can't think straight, which makes it hard to make good decisions; two, you fool yourself into thinking that since you skipped a meal, you can eat whatever you like. Not true.

Jae—While breakfast is a good idea for many people, it's not a good idea for me personally. I don't feel hungry in the morning—I just have my black coffee. What I've noticed is that when I eat breakfast, I think about food more than usual, and it's harder to stick to my plan. I think about what I'm going to eat for lunch and then count down the time until lunch, or think about the snack I want to get right now and then try to convince myself not to get it. The result? There'll be a morning snack, lunch, afternoon snack, more snacks, and eating throughout the day even though I'm not hungry. When I start eating so early in the day, my inner dialogue about food takes up so much mental space—space that I'd rather use to get stuff done.

If you do eat breakfast, make it worth your while: an omelet with veggies, oatmeal with nuts and berries, a fruit and nut yogurt smoothie, or peanut butter on whole grain toast. But please don't start your day at a cereal bar full of refined sugar and other processed carbohydrates!

Snacks: We Can't Live without Them

In many societies around the world (including those where a Mediterranean-type diet is the norm), people do not snack. There's a lot to be said for not snacking, but unfortunately the two of us can't live that way. We need our snacks!

Having said that, snacks can really derail anyone. Some crackers here, a few chips there, a cookie with a spoonful of ice cream chaser— so much junk, so many calories, and so little thought in the process. We've had to change what snacks we eat and where we eat them.

In terms of *where* we eat snacks, it's more a matter of where we *don't* eat them. Neither of us has unhealthy, calorie-dense food near us when we're in the car, at the movies, or watching television. Just those minor changes in our habits have made a *big* difference for us.

Jae—While I try not to snack too much, some days it just can't be avoided like when I have to travel a lot, or I can't make it home to cook dinner for a while after classes or work. When this happens, I turn to high-protein snacks.

Janice—I have to have snacks with me pretty much all the time. I think it's more of an anxiety thing than a hunger thing—but whatever it is, it's a thing. That means I need to prepare ahead of time so I don't go down a rabbit hole of mindlessness, poor choices, and self-recrimination.

We Make Healthy Food Swaps

Food swaps can make a big difference in easing you into pleasurable, healthy eating. We get that steamed broccoli is not a "swap" for coconut cream pie, but we do have some ideas that may help you.

Jae—Sometimes, ordering a pizza and eating the whole thing sounds like an 11 out of 10 idea, but I know it's not going to make me feel good or help me accomplish my goals. When this happens, I know I'm usually craving the taste of the hot tomato sauce and cheese rather than a pizza itself. Luckily, I might have some portabella mushroom caps in the fridge, as well as tomato sauce and cheese, so I can make mushroom cap pizzas. Making the swap will help me avoid eating impulsively or feeling deprived, and I'll feel proud of my success.

Janice—Jae's "portabella pizza" swap drives the point home that it's important to have healthy food available on hand in the kitchen so you can make delicious, healthy choices whenever you need it.

In the recipe section of this book, we have lists of snacks and swaps. Check them out!

Secret #3: We Don't Put Ourselves Last

We wholeheartedly acknowledge that to create and sustain these new healthy-eating habits requires an investment in time and effort. That investment won't be worth it unless you believe *you* are a worthwhile investment.

We've talked before about paradigm shifts. Here are some self-care possibilities for you:

Old Paradigm	New Paradigm
I'll keep chips in the house for my husband and kids.	I don't want to tempt myself unfairly. My family and I will all eat healthier snacks at home.
I'll go to bed two hours late so I can bake a birthday cake for a coworker.	I'll buy a cake at the store on my way to work tomorrow.
I'll go to the gym if I have time.	I deserve to make time to take care of myself.

Your health and well-being are not a selfish luxury—they are the key to being your best self in your family, your job, and your world. Please move yourself from the bottom of your list of priorities. You deserve more, and you'll have so much more to offer others if you take good care of yourself.

List #12: What are the Secrets to Your Success?

As you continue on your new journey, you will discover your own secrets and tricks. Be sure to write them down so you can refer back to them in the future as your relationship with food continues to become more positive and joyful.

STEP NINE:

Hold on to a Good Thing

CHAPTER 23

Keeping Track of Your Progress

> The number on the scale does
> not determine your worth or your
> strength or even your beauty.

L et's review where you are so far in this process. You've created a
list of reasons why you want to change the way you eat. You have
a list of goals to help keep you focused and motivated. You have an
understanding of the healthiest foods to eat and how to incorporate
those foods into your life. You're planning ahead to minimize the
potential for random, unexpected, unhealthy choices. Your kitchen
is looking different, organized in such a way to facilitate your success.
All of this adds up to something we hope you recognize as incredible:
you have taken your relationship with food into your own hands,
and you are much more in control of something that once seemed
to have diabolical control over you. As you continue making these
changes, we recommend tracking your progress in a way that will
keep you honest and, more important, motivated.

Experts in behavioral therapy say a key element in successful weight
loss includes self-monitoring, such as keeping a record of what you

eat, the number of calories, and the number of minutes you spend doing physical activity.[1] In this chapter, we'll discuss some commonly used tools to track your progress, such as calorie counting, measuring body weight, and recording physical activity. We also want to make it clear that these are by no means the only ways to evaluate your progress, and they are not mutually exclusive. Feel free to try several strategies at the same time, or none at all. Remember that the point of monitoring tools is to provide structure and feedback to help you, not shame you, tear you down, or threaten to make you feel disappointed in yourself. They should inspire confidence and give you control.

Should You Count Calories?

Well, it depends. For some people, calorie counting really, really helps. If you are starting out, calorie counting is a great way to have a structured, regimented system that will help you plan ahead and stay accountable; you can then ease back once you feel more successful and confident. For others, counting calories can feel overly stressful, frustrating, and time-consuming. If you have a prior history of an eating disorder, especially one with a restrictive component, calorie counting may be an unwise decision—it may trigger a relapse, which is the last thing we want to happen to you.

Jae—Calorie counting was integral to my personal strategy because I had no concept of food composition or portion size. Before I decided to lose weight, all I knew was that I ate what I wanted when I wanted, and I was gaining twenty pounds a year on average. I did not know how to intuitively eat or moderate my food intake for the day. But I did know how to read a nutritional label; I knew how to add numbers; and I knew how to structure my day. Calorie counting was my salvation, allowing me to calculate my daily caloric allotment based on my height, current weight, and activity level.

I remember the first time I logged my calories for a meal. I ate two bagels slathered in cream cheese, some scrambled eggs, and sausage for breakfast. I calculated the total calories consumed, which was over a thousand. That was just one meal! It was the wake-up call I needed to become aware of the food I was putting in my body. It taught me that there are nearly a hundred calories in a (pathetically small) tablespoon of peanut butter or that I could add as much broccoli as I wanted to my stir-fry for basically no additional calories. Calorie counting helped me understand portion sizes—that a "serving size" of peanut butter was not however many spoonfuls it took until I was sick of it. It gave me structure and a concrete number to work toward; it was a rule that I, as a goal-oriented person, could adhere to. Of course, I was rarely spot-on, but I was close enough, and this set me up for success.

Today, calorie counting remains my primary tool for weight maintenance because I still do not have a perfect brain-stomach communication channel. Calorie counting is great for meal planning because it allows me to be flexible. If I decide I want a piece of chocolate during lunch, I input it in my calorie counting app, where it remains as a non-emotionally-charged number in my log instead of as a "bad" food in my brain. This way, I am not "failing;" I have simply made a rational and predetermined choice, and I'm not disappointed in myself.

MyFitnessPal is a wonderful tool for counting calories, and it can divide large batches of food into individual portions. When I first started, I also used a food scale to calculate exactly how much of each food was going into each portion, which helped me to avoid over- or underestimating how many calories I was actually consuming.

Janice*—I'm in the counting group, too. It helps me stay honest. I do not count the calories in non-starchy vegetables and fruits. I'm confident that I'll never, ever have a weight or health problem by replacing cookies with cantaloupe. I'll be healthier, and I won't go hungry.*

Essentially, we both calorie count, but to different degrees. We each do what works for us, and we encourage you to find your style.

Should You Weigh Yourself?

Before we jump in, here are two important things to consider when weighing yourself. First, you are not a number. The number on the scale does not determine your worth or your strength or even your beauty. Second, if you have a "history" with the scale and find yourself having an obsessive relationship with it, put it away. Don't allow yourself to go down that slippery, dark slope.

If you want to weigh yourself, should it be once a week? Every day? There are different ways to approach it, so decide what works best for you. Some people like to weigh themselves once a week so they can see the general trend and make sure they're heading in the right direction, which clues them in on whether they need to make substantive changes to how they're eating and moving. This is a more relaxed approach that appeals to people who get discouraged by the minimal day-to-day changes or who have a prior history with eating disorders and obsessive behaviors. Other people like to weigh themselves every day because it helps them with accountability. Seeing their weight each morning motivates them to make better food choices during the day.

Janice—*Personally, I think that weighing yourself only once a week can be deceiving. If you've eaten a salty meal the night before you get on the scale, it might register a higher weight than what is really reflective of your progress, which can be both discouraging and misleading. Plus, you won't know what's going on for a whole additional week.*

Jae—*I went back to weighing myself daily when I got closer to my goal weight and saw that my progress was slowing down. I wanted to keep myself more accountable, and I liked having a day-by-day idea of how my weight was trending. However, I eventually found myself feeling obsessive about my weight and my body and recognized that it was an unhealthy mindset, so I went back to weighing myself weekly. But just because this happened to me doesn't mean it will happen to you! It's definitely possible to weigh yourself every day and not have it become a compulsion.*

Whatever system you choose, do not weigh yourself more than once a day. The body changes throughout the day, especially with added food weight and water retention. It's misleading, and it will make you obsessed and crazy. If weighing yourself does little more than provoke anxiety, then maybe it isn't for you at all.

Tracking Physical Activity: Get Credit for Every Step You Take

We've talked about the usefulness of setting goals throughout this book, and it is certainly true for exercise. Activity monitors can assist with tracking your progress toward those goals, whether it be counting steps, burning calories, or measuring time spent on various types of exercise.

Jae—I recommend tracking your physical activity because you will have a reference to look back on to evaluate your progress. This can be really motivating if you ever hit a rut and need some inspiration. There's always the reliable pen and paper method—I know many people who do powerlifting and just keep track of everything in a notebook. It's simple, you have complete control over the structure of it, and it can change with your needs. The downside is it can be potentially time-consuming to figure out what format you need, but once you have a layout that works, your time will be greatly reduced.

No matter what you think about technology, it has arguably become a valuable tool for keeping track of exercise. There are a seemingly infinite number of apps out there that can help you. I have used trial and error with many apps to figure out which ones have features that work best for me. But remember that what works for me may not always work for you. Here are the criteria I use to decide what apps are likely to be useful to me:

1. *It's easy to use. How is the user interface? Is it easy to figure out? Do I like how it looks? If it's not intuitive, I'm just going to get frustrated and will not use it, which defeats the purpose.*
2. *It tracks what I need. I like to run, so when I search for new running apps to try out, I look for things like whether I can customize the time cues, whether there is an integrated training program, and whether the map is accurate when it comes to calculating distance.*
3. *It helps me measure progress. Many of the apps I like to use will tell me at the end of a run whether or not it was my fastest time or a new distance record. I find this motivating as I can see that I'm getting better.*

For running, I like MapMyRun, which is integrated with MyFitnessPal. Since I've used it for so long, it contains a lot of my running history and has become very intuitive. I also use Nike Run Club for the half marathon I'm training for right now. It has a training plan that takes into account how quickly I want to complete the race, how long I have to prepare for the race, and some other goals. It creates a plan for me that will change if I miss runs or if I'm running faster or slower than anticipated. I like the way this app is set up because it doesn't make me feel bad if I miss a run or if I'm not exactly hitting the goal it has set up for my training. Because of this, I'm more likely to stick with it.

When it comes to weight lifting, I have found that a notebook or my own custom-made spreadsheet on Excel has worked best for tracking my lifting progress. I can put in the different lifts and accessory lifts that I work on; plus, it's free. I like the flexibility of this method, and I have the ease of changing it up whenever I need to.

Portion Control: Good Idea or Just Another Form of Deprivation?

Americans tend to eat huge portions of food. All-you-can-eat buffets have great appeal, even though the food is usually mediocre at best. People go to the movies and get enough soda and popcorn to feed everyone in their row of seats. Having said that, being on a diet where portions are strictly limited is, for most people, anxiety-provoking and unsustainable.

Janice—"Portion control," to me, sounds like I'm being controlled and not allowed to eat enough. Using the typical "diet" model, this means deprivation, which ultimately means failure. I'm a high-volume eater. If I think that I'm not going to eat enough to feel satisfied, I'm going to feel anxious, unhappy, and unwilling to repeat that experience. Maybe that's why intuitive eating doesn't work for me. My intuition points me in the way of grilled cheese sandwiches and endless Hershey's Kisses.

As I've said in Chapter 22, at every meal, I eat all my vegetables first in order to get a little full, to let my brain have awareness of that fullness, and to buy some time before I move on to the more calorie-dense foods. Also, I find that if I start out with, say, one piece of chicken, I'll want a second piece of chicken instead of the broccoli. By starting with the broccoli, and by eating a lot of it, I've guaranteed myself that I've put the healthiest, lowest-calorie food in my belly first. And by then, a single piece of chicken doesn't feel like "portion control;" it just feels like enough.

Jae—Once I've eaten a lot of vegetables, space in my stomach has been taken up and my brain has a fighting chance to register that I'm starting to feel full. After that, it's so much easier to limit portions of other foods. Also, planning what I'm going to eat ahead of time is a godsend because it allows me eat in a calm and controlled way. Planning portion size in advance is so helpful for me as I still have an issue with portion control. It takes impulse out of the equation, which has been integral to my success.

Our model says that you do not eat unlimited calorie-dense foods, such as beans and nuts (even though they're really healthy) if you want to lose weight. However, notice that we say *do not* instead of *cannot*. The choice is still yours.

Let's say you're at a restaurant, and you're served an enormous portion of food (that is not steamed vegetables). You might feel like eating all of it because you "hate wasting food," but that's just not a valid argument. If you habitually clean your overflowing plate, there's a good chance you're increasing your risk of diabetes, heart disease, stroke, cancer, and arthritis—and you're still not going to save any starving children. If you don't want to waste food, you can simply take some home for later. If you can't take home the extra food, then you just don't.

Eating more food than you need in one sitting isn't good for you or anyone else. You're not responsible for the amount of food someone serves you, and eating more than you want or need is not "getting your money's worth." In fact, think about the money you'll be saving by eating in a healthy way and not needing to buy medication for diabetes or high blood pressure later on!

There is one easy, proven way of controlling portions: use smaller plates, bowls, and glasses for less unhealthy foods. Using smaller plates tricks your brain—and your stomach—into thinking you have a larger portion. It has been found that you actually do want more and eat more when your food is served on larger plates and your drinks in larger glasses.[2]

Progress Pictures

Jae—I'm a visual person, and progress pictures were one of the big reasons I stayed on track. Taking my first picture, my "before" picture, was one of the hardest things I've ever done. It was painful. I took photos from the front, side, and back, saved and dated them, and hid them deep in folders on my computer. Having to face my exposed body was like encountering my biggest insecurity. However, I knew that those photos would be the last ones I would ever take feeling that way about myself. I knew, from that point on, that every picture I would take would show me looking healthier and leave me feeling more inspired and confident in myself.

These pictures were incredibly helpful when I hit my motivational ruts, when I would think to myself, "Why am I even doing this? I've made all the right choices but nothing is working; I'll never change." Pulling out my progress pictures and setting them side by side one another was evidence that my body was really changing. I couldn't argue with a picture.

I took measurements, too. When I started preparing for the Couch to 5K Program (C25K), beginning at a level of no exercise and working up to successfully running the full race, I was frustrated because I lost only eight pounds after the entire six weeks—but I also lost almost ten inches from my waist! My body changed way more dramatically than what was reflected by the scale. Having those pictures and measurements were a large source of validation and motivation. I've reached a point where I feel proud to take a progress picture of my body, and it's exciting to know that I'm still changing!

CHAPTER 24

Sustaining Weight Loss— The Secrets to Our Success

> One candy bar doesn't "ruin" the day. One day of crazy eating doesn't "ruin" the week. You're not a failure.

The two of us are among only 20 percent of people who have successfully achieved long-term weight loss.[1, 2] Before we talk about our strategies for success, first, here is a summary of common denominators for almost all people who have maintained healthy weight loss:[3]

- A relatively low-calorie, low-glycemic-load diet with adequate protein
- Regular physical activity, an average of 30 to 60 minutes a day of moderate-intensity exercise
- Consistent monitoring, particularly of weight and caloric intake
- Mental strategies

There are many factors, both internal and external, that contribute to the difficulty of maintaining weight loss.

Internal Factors

The Body's Response to Weight Loss

It's simple, and it's sad: when you lose weight, your energy requirements go down as well, which means you need to consume fewer calories in order to sustain weight loss.[4] As if that's not bad enough, hormonal changes occur in the body that may actually increase your appetite.[5, 6]

The Brain's Response to Weight Loss

Once you've lost weight, the scale doesn't continue to go down, you don't get to wear smaller sizes, and people no longer marvel at your new appearance. With this new status quo, there's bound to be some letdown. It's not surprising that so many people experience "behavioral fatigue."[7] In addition, as the body continues to need fewer calories and your appetite doesn't compensate for that need, it's easy to blame yourself for having gotten "lazy" or not having enough "willpower" anymore. How easy it is, then, to view yourself as a failure and to just give up.

External Factors

Unhealthy Food Is Everywhere

We've discussed—even demonized—highly processed, inexpensive, hyper-delicious processed foods. These crave-worthy, calorie-dense foods are ubiquitous, and they easily undermine your efforts to lose weight and to maintain weight loss.[8, 9]

Misguided Health Care Professionals (That Means You, Too, Janice)

As we explained, physiologic changes in the body will cause you to need fewer calories, but they will not decrease your appetite enough to compensate for that change. Why, then, do some doctors persist in telling you that it's a "simple equation" of calories in versus calories out? Why do doctors reinforce your notion that you just need more willpower?[10] We'll discuss this in detail in the next chapter.

The Keys to Successfully Maintaining Weight Loss

Criticism from your family members, dire warnings from your doctor, and even financial incentives may all provide some motivation for you to try to lose weight, but only in the short term,[11] and we hate the short term. After all, if you go back to your unhealthy habits, you'll just feel more frustrated and pessimistic than ever. On the other hand, *sustained* weight loss is possible when you develop your own strategies that are meaningful and enjoyable enough for you to stick with them and continue your self-directed motivation.

Key One: Smart Eating Matters

For starters, stay on your low-glycemic-load diet.[12] In particular, foods that are high in fiber will fill you up and prevent you from feeling hungry soon after you eat. Increasing the amount of protein you eat also has a satiating effect[13]—you need increase to your protein intake by just five percent to have that effect.[14] Plant proteins, particularly from beans, nuts, and legumes, are associated with the greatest benefit.[15] Fish and Greek yogurt are additional versatile and healthy sources of protein.[16]

Another factor related to smart eating is the timing of calorie consumption, as we talked about in Chapter 4. Relatively larger breakfasts and smaller dinners are associated with greater initial weight loss[17] and higher maintenance rates.[18]

Key Two: Smart Moving Matters

Once you weigh less, your body adapts and needs fewer calories to maintain the lower weight.[19] Your slimmer body simply requires less fuel to keep it going. Additionally, some people's bodies adapt to weight loss by making them hungrier.[20, 21]

To keep on track, you need to eat less. But you're already eating so much less! What's the solution to revving up your metabolism? Exercise. While physical activity doesn't have a large role in *initial* weight loss, at least compared to decreasing caloric intake, exercise is essential in *maintaining* weight loss.[22] An average of 30 to 60 minutes per day of physical activity is recommended. In a nutshell, **"After weight loss, physical activity is a major determinant in the prevention of future weight gain."**[23]

If going to the gym is less fun than going to the dentist, then go dancing or walking with a friend. Just keep your body moving!

Key Three: Numbers Matter

As we discussed in the last chapter, when you're trying to *lose* weight, there are pros and cons with monitoring tools, such as weighing yourself and counting calories. In order to *maintain* weight loss, however, the pros definitely win out—self-monitoring is highly effective.[24] There's lots of evidence showing that people who maintain weight loss have in common weighing themselves at least three times a week, recording their food and caloric intake, and counting the number of minutes per day of physical activity.[25]

We have both discovered how easy it was, once we stopped weighing ourselves regularly, for the weight to creep back on. So we're sticking to the more disciplined approach. But there's a caveat: make sure to balance out the discipline with understanding and kindness!

Key Four: Support Matters

Call a friend when you think you might go down the rabbit hole of comfort food. Find an exercise buddy or group so you'll feel accountable to be active even when the couch looks like a better idea. Don't worry about "bothering" people. When someone sincerely asks you for help, doesn't it usually make you feel good to come to their aid?

Key Five, Six, Seven . . . and a Hundred: Taking Care of Yourself Matters

Don't Go Back to Beating Yourself Up

A pint of mint chocolate chip ice cream can make you feel oh-so-much better, right? Yes—for five minutes. And then the self-recrimination, the disgust, and the shame set in.

Your old coping mechanisms for dealing with stress, anger, sadness, and other emotions did not work. Comfort eating does not offer comfort, and stress eating does not relieve stress. More than half of the people who regain weight identify depression and anxiety as triggers for emotional eating. The people who were most successful in keeping weight off were those who continued to use "dietary restraint."[26] In other words, they continued to eat healthy foods, and they continued to eat only when they were *physically* hungry.

Along with the discipline of eating healthy, non-processed foods; being physically active; and monitoring the numbers, there's something else of equal importance: kindness. Ultimately, it's not about the weight, really, as much as it's about feeling good physically, feeling confident emotionally, and feeling deserving of taking care of yourself.

Remember, You're Already Ahead of the Game

If you've lost weight in a healthy way, then you have already developed new coping skills. They're still effective—don't abandon them! Go back to what worked for you in the first place. Review the lists you made and the habits you've changed. Think about the effective ways you've learned to respond to stressful situations. Ramp up your mindfulness and positive self-talk. You've already developed these skills, and you've proven to yourself that you are disciplined, motivated, and committed to living a more vibrant, shame-free life. Now it's time to apply your strategies and mindset to this new challenge. It's a challenge without an endpoint; it's a new way of life. A life of health, vitality, and confidence.

Relapses Happen. That's Okay.

Dietary lapses and relapses aren't just possible—they're inevitable. Old coping strategies die hard, and the desire to turn to food in times of stress, anger, and sadness runs deep. You're not perfect—so join the club. What matters is what happens next. One candy bar doesn't "ruin" the day. One day of crazy eating doesn't "ruin" the week. You're not a failure.

Sure, successful long-term weight loss entails preventing backslides as much as possible, but sometimes you can't—or you just don't. The important thing is not to submit to pessimism and self-loathing. You've already invested so much, so don't abandon your healthy approach to living. Just as important as the strategies you used to lose the weight is the mindset you need to have now—a mindset comprised of self-compassion, optimism, confidence, and a sense of self-worth—which can help you get right back on track if you slip. As much as the weight loss itself, we're willing to bet that the process of self-care and the concept of self-worth are what has made you feel great.

Employ all of these resources of mindfulness, kindness, and reframing that you've learned, and now change the paradigm:

Old paradigm	New paradigm
I just ate cake and blew it. Once again, I'm a failure.	I wish I hadn't chosen to eat cake when I was stressed. Now, I'm going to make good choices for the rest of the day, and I'm going to prep a salad for tomorrow.

Jae—Especially when I first started changing the way I ate, I slipped up a lot in terms of not eating what I was meant to be eating. I was not perfect! However, it helped me to view each mistake as just that—a mistake. I didn't say, "Oh shoot, now it's back to square one." Instead of giving up, even for the rest of that one day, I said, "Oops, I messed up," and simply went right back to trying to eat the foods that were right for me. I was in this for the long haul, and I wasn't going to let one mistake derail me.

Do a Cost-Benefit Analysis

There are times when the costs of continued disciplined eating and disciplined physical activity seem high—maybe too high. But what was the cost of not being able to keep up physically with your family? What was the cost of the misery you felt after a binge-eating episode? What was the cost of feeling simultaneously invisible and hyper-visible?

Weight loss and maintaining weight loss are associated with "both striving to achieve positive outcomes (promotion) and striving to avoid negative outcomes (prevention)."[27] For losing weight, the promotion approach is the most effective; whereas for maintenance, it's prevention.[28] Prevention consists of taking steps to prevent reverting to feeling less confident and less worthy, along with avoiding dealing with disease, discomfort, or lack of mobility. The point is that both systems—promotion and prevention—work, sometimes one more than the other. Use them both to keep on track.

Whatever system or systems you use, here's something to consider: "*Current* feelings of eating-associated or weight-associated shame are associated with increased caloric intake. Feelings related to *anticipated* shame associated with overeating, on the other hand, are associated with decreased caloric intake."[29] Ditch what has become the habitual, instantaneous shame associated with eating. Instead, try to think *ahead* of time about how you'll feel after you eat the apple pie (perhaps remorseful) instead of the apple (proud of yourself).

We get it—it's *hard* to keep going once the headiness of weight loss is over. We both love eating sweets and sitting on the couch watching Netflix, and sometimes it seems that it would be so easy to go back to these old habits. So, in addition to needing to maintain discipline, we also have to maintain a constant refrain: **this new path is what I truly want for my body, my brain, my emotions, and my future.**

Janice—One of my patients created a "fitness vision board," complete with photographs, aphorisms, and fitness challenges. I love this idea because it reinforces the concept of an ongoing, lifelong, healthy approach to food and activity.

By ending the deprivation mindset and instead fixing your attention on the good stuff, you're able to take the negative thoughts about what you've had to give up and reframe them in such a way that you can focus on the benefits, which are enormous.

Most important, you've already reaped so many benefits because of the changes you made—and you did them yourself. You figured out strategies that worked. There's no reason you can't figure out strategies to avoid regaining the weight. The people who are able to remain confident and positive about their progress and who are able to develop strategies are the people who are least likely to regain weight.

Continue Finding Ways to Stay Motivated

Jae—*Many people have asked me how I was able to keep motivated over the course of five years. First, I want to point out that my journey may have started five years ago, but it is still very real and continuous. I now know I can't go back to spending my whole day sitting in bed or eating half a pizza if I want to seriously maintain the changes I have made in order to honor my body.*

However, I must admit it is harder to maintain weight than to lose weight. I was able to sustain weight loss for just over twenty-four continuous months, and the following three years have proven to be way more difficult than I ever could have anticipated. I was so used to being meticulous about my calories and exercise in order to sustain my weight loss in the early stages that when I stopped being meticulous, I gained some weight. I also didn't understand that I needed to ingest fewer calories, which led to more weight gain. Not a lot, but enough to feel bad about it. The weight gain is difficult because I sometimes catch myself in the mindset where I think, I'm going to get fat again. *But here's the thing—I have already done so much to change my relationship with food that it's not possible for me to ever return to that point again. So, while weight gain is not ideal, I know that whatever I have gained I will know how to lose it again. I will be okay. That's what has worked for me, and I'm confident you can find a successful path for yourself, too.*

STEP TEN:

Have a Goal of Vibrancy, Not Thinness

CHAPTER 25

Will You Ever Be Thin Enough? Should That Even Be a Question?

> You are not a thin person stuck inside a fat person. You are a person.

These are very difficult questions to ask in a fat-shaming culture.

- We are ashamed of ourselves for being overweight.
- We judge others for being overweight, and we're ashamed of feeling that way.
- We want others to be ashamed of themselves for judging us.
- None of this is working.

Our society makes it really, *really* difficult for overweight people to feel good about themselves. And that makes this chapter really, *really* difficult for us to write. We have written this entire book with the goal of encouraging you to take care of yourself on every level and to feel good about yourself **right now**. How can you stop feeling shame when it seems like the rest of the world *wants* you to be ashamed?

It takes mental toughness to counter that attitude from others. How do you maintain your sense of self-worth when you're consistently and cruelly undervalued because of the pervasive stigma in our society against obesity? Perhaps the worst part about bias against obese people is that, unlike other forms of bias, it is actually *socially acceptable.* The bias comes from all sides: family, peers, teachers, the media, and potential employers and partners. Obese people are often perceived as lazy, undisciplined, and unmotivated.[1, 2, 3] How can there possibly be helpful responses? Actually, we do think they exist, but first, let's talk about the challenges.

Bias Starts Early

Bias starts early and lasts a lifetime. The cruelty may begin in childhood. Obese children are subject to bullying, the detrimental effects of which often last throughout adulthood.[4] They are more likely to skip school because of the emotional abuse they suffer and are less likely to have friends.[5] Teachers, not just other children, contribute to this dreadful situation.[6] Not surprisingly, adolescents who endure negative comments about their weight are more likely to be obese and to engage in disordered eating habits as adults.

Who are the most likely people to shame children about their weight? The answer: their parents.[7] Many obese adults say that their parents' weight-shaming comments to them when they were children, often veiled as "constructive criticism" or "harmless teasing" or even "encouragement," are a major contributor to their lifelong shame about their bodies and their unhealthy relationship with food.

We should add here that parents of children with (or without) obesity usually care deeply about their children's well-being. They genuinely want to help their children, but they may be communicating in a way that is counterproductive and even traumatizing.

Bias Continues Throughout Life

This weight bias has terrible ramifications in the personal lives of many obese people. They may have less of a sense of emotional well-being and often experience more rejection in dating contexts. This is especially true for women.

The stigma goes even further than that. Educational and occupational opportunities are unfairly limited. Obese people are less likely to be admitted to graduate school programs and are less likely to be hired and promoted. They are stigmatized by the media. They are more likely to suffer from depression and anxiety.[8, 9]

In other words, weight bias has terrible ramifications with regard to academic achievement, financial success, and emotional well-being throughout life. To make matters worse, one of the ways that obesity differs from other forms of stigma is that overweight people tend to be biased against *one another*,[10, 11] making it a particularly isolating and lonely situation.

Doctor, Heal Thyself

Janice—*Forgive me. Until I struggled with weight myself, I didn't have the vaguest idea of how to be helpful to my patients. In fact, I was harmful. If your doctor tells you to eat less and exercise more, that implies you don't already know that; it implies you don't care; it implies you just need to try harder. Are you ever again going to trust that doctor as a person who might be able to really help you with your challenges? Why should you, when all she has done is to pile on even more shame?*

Until I gained weight myself, I just didn't get it. But boy, did that ever change! I'm grateful to my patients for letting me enter into a dialogue with them where I can offer support and encouragement. With each of my patients, we look at her individual challenges and create an individual set of goals and strategies. My suggestions may work, or maybe they won't. Goals and strategies change. The important things, however, do not change: there is no judgment or blame or failure. There are only difficulties that are followed by new opportunities. It is all positive. Clearly, to my great distress, I'm not the only doctor who was clueless.

Traditionally, most physicians think that obesity is basically a behavioral problem related to nothing more complicated than eating too much and exercising too little. Like other members of our society, doctors and medical students are biased toward obese people[12] and characterize them as "noncompliant, lacking in motivation and self-indulgent."[13] Instead of addressing the patient's needs and concerns, physicians are all too willing to blame every problem on weight and to blame the patient for being in this predicament. In Roxane Gay's memoir, *Hunger*, she makes an observation that unfortunately applies to doctors: "When people use the word 'obese,' they aren't merely being literal. They are offering forth an accusation."[14]

Jae—Before I lost weight, I was so embarrassed to go to the doctor. I used to absolutely dread stepping on the scale and seeing the little shake of the head from my nurse as she filled out my chart and said, "Oh, just a little higher up from last time, dear." Like I wasn't aware.

The doctor was even worse—the only thing she saw was my fat. I felt dehumanized. She automatically saw my obesity as an explanation for any and all symptoms I had. Then she would lecture me on the importance of diet and exercise.

Of course I knew I was fat; I'm not stupid. I knew my weight was a significant problem because I was the one living with it. I knew how crappy I felt, how sluggish and tired I always was. She didn't have to tell me that. It's so demoralizing and hurtful when you go in to see someone who has sworn to heal you, and instead, they make you feel as if you are being judged or viewed as "lesser" just for your weight status. All I wanted was for her to see beyond my fat, to not devalue me as a human being, and to genuinely try to help me.

Janice—*Overweight women have an increased risk of cervical cancer, too. Now that's particularly heartbreaking to me. Cervical cancer is related to a virus; weight should have nothing to do with it. But studies have showed that overweight women are less likely to seek preventive care, even after controlling for socioeconomic status.*[15] *Women who do not get regular Pap testing are at a much, much greater risk for developing cervical cancer than those who do. And why do overweight women not get regular Pap testing? I think it's because they feel so much shame about their bodies and because they don't want to endure further shaming at a doctor's office. So, they just stay home.*

Actually, You're Even Worse to Yourself than Doctors Are

Janice—*My dear friend Amy is my hero. When she and her boyfriend were once getting ready to go to a party, she asked him, "How do I look?" He answered, "That dress looks a little tight." Here's why Amy is my hero: although she was embarrassed and hurt, she had enough self-esteem to recognize the hurtfulness of his comment and to call him out on it. I don't know that I would have had that same response. I might have berated myself for being fat. I might have put on my pajamas and stayed home.*

The most severe damage caused by weight stigma is actually *internalized* bias, the unjustified criticism that you heap on yourself. Internalized weight bias, which refers to the acceptance overweight people have about the society's unfair and untrue stereotypes and negative beliefs about them, is more damaging than all the forms of bias that come from the outside. Internalized bias is completely understandable, of course. You live in a fat-shaming culture, and you're a part of the culture, too. It's not surprising that you would come to believe the negative stereotypes that are so prevalent. It's crucial to understand, though, that blaming yourself may actually be a source of even greater unhappiness and low self-esteem than the bias that's aimed at you from the outside world.[16]

Let us be clear: perhaps someone said something intentionally hurtful about your weight when you were a child. It wasn't okay for them to talk to you like that then, and it's not okay for you to talk to yourself like that now.

Janice—Medical school was a very happy time of my life. I felt like I was doing something worthwhile, and I was proud to be there. I loved school, and I loved my classmates. So why did I miss my twenty-year reunion? It was because I weighed forty pounds more than I had in med school, and I was embarrassed and ashamed. I can't say with assurance that I would never let myself make that decision again. Even as I write these words, I think to myself, "What is wrong with this person?" I'm upset with myself for not being strong enough to be more than a mere product of my culture, but there you have it.

Judging Yourself Leads to Judging Others

One of the most insidious and harmful consequences of internalized bias is that it "legitimizes" fat-shaming others. We criticize and judge others because of their size, all the while reserving our harshest judgment for ourselves. We have both struggled with internalizing the cultural norms that dictate how people should look.

Jae—When I went for job interviews, I was sure people were judging me. I thought that because I judged them, too. When I was in college, if I saw a professor who was overweight, I thought they were doing something wrong, like me, even though I knew they were normal people with normal priorities. I hate feeling like that about other people, and I hate knowing that people once thought the same way about me.

Well, this is all kind of depressing. But help is on the way. Here are some ideas that may be useful to you:

Stop Fat-Shaming Yourself

This is key. You deserve to be loved by others and by yourself right now. Your weight has nothing to do with your worth. Yes, that's a hard truth to hold on to when your worth is being unfairly diminished. In this sense, though, the fact that internalized bias is the most damaging form of bias is comforting—because it means you have some control! You don't have to try to take on the entire culture in which you live; just take on your own prejudices. Yes, weight consciousness and body positivity can coexist.

If you think that you're not a good enough person now and that you will be worthy of love and respect only after you lose weight, please rethink your strategy. Self-loathing is guaranteed to lead to more shame and more weight or even an eating disorder, where you're never "thin" enough. Look back all the way to Chapter 2: the antidote to shame is kindness. Be kind to yourself—not dishonest, but kind. When you think something terrible about yourself, try to catch yourself in the act and replace that thought—*reframe* that thought—with something more positive. Do this because, if nothing else, please know that **no one succeeds with sustainable weight loss through self-hatred.** We talked about this earlier in the book: before you shed even a single pound, if you can let go of the shame, then you will be able to carry out a strategy that will *result in sustainable weight loss.*

Interestingly, hurling invective toward those who've hurt you seems not to work, either. Positive strategies such as compassionate self-talk and seeking support from others is associated with higher self-acceptance and self-esteem. On the other hand, negative strategies, such as retorts aimed at offending parties, are actually associated with more depression.[17] We have both tried changing our bodies by hating our bodies and ourselves. Guess what? It didn't work.

Stop Fat-Shaming Others, Especially Kids

Please, please do not be critical toward your kids about their weight. We owe it to our children to not only feed them nourishing, healthy food, but also stop the fat-shaming that starts so young. What kind of society is it where nine-year-olds (many of whom are not even overweight) are "on a diet"? You know all too well how shame has affected you. We urge you to stress positive habits and activities, as opposed to belittling, guilt-inducing, negative forms of "motivation." Words matter, and we recommend talking about healthy eating and movement. More than that, we recommend *modeling* healthy eating and movement yourself. And, speaking of words, saying fewer negative things out loud about yourself is such a gift to your children, too. They will become much less likely to internalize those thoughts and words and carry that burden themselves, and we'll talk more about this in Chapter 27. Let's first begin with ourselves to turn from shame toward compassion and kindness.

Janice—*I love how one of my patients was able to reframe the shaming she'd endured as a child: "My mother said I was an ugly duckling. I've decided to be a swan."*

Jae—*I did not lose weight until I came to that decision myself. A relative once told me, "I'll give you ten dollars for every pound you lose." When they said that, I felt hurt and devalued. I was stubborn and rebellious when people told me I needed to lose weight. I knew full well that being obese was unhealthy for me, but when others gave me orders, it did not help. I did not feel their concern for me or their desire to see me have a better life; I felt like they did not like me for who I was, which fed the negative emotional cycle. I only started to lose weight when I wanted to do so for myself. When I wanted to live differently. When I wanted to make a sustainable lifestyle change.*

Appreciate What Your Body Is Doing for You

It is time to reframe the way you think about your body. Your criticism isn't fair to you, it's not helpful, and it minimizes everything that's positive about your physical self. One of the reasons so many people engage in yo-yo dieting is because of the distress they feel when they haven't lost "enough" weight or still don't look "good enough."[18] How about *reframing* something negative you said about your body that's more positive and loving—and probably more correct?

First, move from "I hate my body" to "I love what my body can do." Do you have to love your body? That's up to you. But surely, you can appreciate what it's doing for you *right now*. Your brain and eyes work—here you are, reading. Your body works—it got you out of bed this morning. You can take it from there, toward moving in the direction of love.

You'll be better able to appreciate your body if you take better care of it. One of the best ways to do this is to move more. Regardless of what they actually weigh, victims of weight bias exercise less.[19] That's not surprising. In Chapter 15, we discussed how engaging in physical exercise can feel particularly daunting for overweight people because of the judgment they feel from others. Once again, though, studies show that the judgment from yourself may be more damaging than judgment from others.[20, 21] So, try being less judgmental about yourself, and let your body move more.

In journalist and author Lindy West's provocative, hilarious, painful book, *Shrill*, she writes, "Maybe you are thin. You hiked that trail and you are fit and beautiful and wanted . . . and I'm miles behind you, my breathing ragged. But you didn't carry this up the mountain. You only carried yourself. How hard would you breathe if you had to carry me? You couldn't. But I can."[22] What a brilliant example of how to reframe your attitude toward your body!

What, then, can we finally say about this tension between accepting one's body and striving to be thinner? Perhaps it's simply this: being obese may be unhealthy, but it's not a moral failing, and we all share in the responsibility to detach shame from body size. You do not deserve to be in solitary confinement.

Janice—*Here's what I tell my patients: I don't care what you weigh. I care that you eat healthy food and that you incorporate movement into your life. I care that you don't hate yourself. I care that you get enough sleep. I care that you spend time with people you love. I care that you go to the dentist twice a year and practice safe sex. The rest is up to you.*

Your body is not enemy territory.
Your body has not betrayed you.
You are not a thin person stuck inside a fat person. You are a person.
You are alive. Savor that today, and move forward with optimism.

CHAPTER 26

Jae, 140 Pounds Later

> You are not a thin person stuck
> inside a fat person. You are a person.

Jae—There have been so many wonderful changes since I lost weight. But I need to tell you that I truly believed that losing weight would make everything so much easier, that I would have my life together and all my problems would just go away. This was not even remotely true. I still found ways to scrutinize my body and find imperfections. I still had problems—they were just new ones. It took me a long time—and I'm not all the way there yet—to understand that if you don't find a way to love yourself and who you are, regardless of how your body looks, losing weight is not going to solve the problem. You have to take care of yourself emotionally and mentally as much as you do physically. Coming to this realization was really hard to accept. Making changes was a slow process; and even now, years after losing so much weight and maintaining that weight loss, I'm actively working on changing my mindset in so many ways. The process continues. Let me tell you about some of those changes:

Social Changes

- When I was obese, I was anxious about every social situation. I felt like I was being judged for my fatness, not my personality. This was verified in situations like the countless times guys would come up to me and a friend, only to literally ignore my existence for the remainder of the conversation. The same people who would not give me the time of day when I was obese now contact me via social media to ask how I am and what I've been up to. When I was invisible before, now I am someone who's worth their time. Just because I lost the weight? Just because I fit a societal standard of beauty? This is particularly relevant to men. When people message me to ask what I've been up to or say that they don't recognize me, while flattering, I still view that remark as, "Now you're worth my time." I was worth your time five years ago, so bug off.

- Men now walk up to me and ask me to smile. No, I do not appreciate this unwelcome attention and obnoxious behavior. I feel uncomfortable and violated. I'll smile when I want to; I will not smile when some jerk wants me to wear a Happy Face for him.

- I used to worry that if I was eating too much, eating something that wasn't "healthy," or eating too quickly, people would think, "No wonder she's so big." And if I wasn't eating, people would ask if I was on a diet, which was also uncomfortable. Now that I'm a healthy weight, I'm not as embarrassed about food when I'm around other people. I eat what I want when I'm in social situations without being preoccupied with what others might think. This has been a big stress reducer and has taken away so much of my anxiety about social interactions.

- People have told me they think of me as a very fit and active person. I still find this almost laughable—only because I never thought anyone would associate me with those traits in a million years. I've found that people have more positive attitudes toward you if you are physically active.

- I no longer have to—or choose to—let being fat hold me back from doing the things I'm interested in. Instead of staying behind, I join my friends for walks, parties, going out, and socializing in general. I don't have to convince myself to go or muster up the motivation; I just go.

- My sense of humor had to change. Some people cope with their size by making fun of it so they get to be in control of the joke, instead of having a joke made at their expense. Now that I'm a healthy weight, I have had to watch myself when it comes to making jokes or even comments in general that insinuate I am fat, since I'm not fat anymore. There have been awkward instances when I was talking to someone who didn't know my history about what it is like being fat or about the judgment large people face, only to be on the receiving end of a puzzled look, as if they were wondering how I could possibly know what being fat feels like or how I can contribute to that perspective.

- People hit on me a lot more. Before my weight loss, no one flirted with me at all. While I am still pretty oblivious and learning to become aware of the signs, I definitely notice that it's occurring with a higher frequency. It's allowed me to feel more empowered when it comes to interacting with potential romantic partners, since, for the first time, I feel like I can be selective with my partners and commit to my standards for what I want in a potential partner. But I acknowledge that having the luxury of people who are attracted to me allows me be selective. This is a privilege that normal-weight people do not necessarily understand that they have in a fat-shaming culture.

- I feel that people value me more now, compared to when I was obese. This is something I find very hard to deal with because I think that my body size should have nothing to do with who I am as a person and the things I am capable of accomplishing. Before my weight loss, I felt completely invisible. I felt that people did not want to hear what I had to say, that they didn't think I could contribute or be a part of something. This was demoralizing because I was being judged based on one aspect of my appearance, instead of based on who I was. Now that I'm smaller, I feel like people are more patient, more willing to listen to me, and more willing to put stock in my opinions. This could perhaps also be due to the fact that I have more confidence in myself as a part of growing up, but regardless, it's a difference that affects how I interact with others.

- Sometimes, though, people seem to treat me like I'm stupid, perhaps because of the way I dress and the "prettier" aspects of my appearance. I've noticed they actually talk more slowly to me or ask whether I'm sure I want to do X or whether I need help doing Y. Nope, I'm perfectly capable of doing things on my own; I'm no less intelligent just because I look a certain way.

Everyday Differences

- There are people in my life who view my accomplishments as a result of my weight loss, rather than because of the fact that I am hardworking, determined, and strong-willed. Someone said, verbatim, "Wow, you changed your mindset; now look at all the other things coming your way!" They had already been coming my way, and my weight had nothing to do with my ability to succeed.

- I admit I still worry about the possibility of getting fat again, and that occupies a lot of mental space that could be used on other things (like my graduate degree!). I know that it's actually not possible for me to ever get to the point of being fat again, now that I am equipped with the tools and strategies that have changed my relationship with food.

- I used to spend a lot of money on clothes when I was getting bigger and bigger. Then, when I started losing weight, I had to spend money because I was getting smaller and smaller. Now that I'm maintaining my current size, I finally have a stable wardrobe and am able to build a set of clothes that represent my style. When I was obese, I felt like I was not allowed to have a personal style. Instead of wearing clothes that reflected my personality and taste, I had to buy clothes that flattered by body type. My wardrobe consisted of clothing that allowed me to cover my body and feel comfortable in public. I was conscious of every angle and every single article of clothing that I wore. I actively avoided any clothing that had references to food or exercise because I worried about other people's judgment. Stores would not even carry my size, which communicated the notion that people my size were so undesirable they weren't even given a physical space or physical representation. Clothing is not only supposed to reflect your personality, it is also an extension of yourself and your identity. Clothing is something we use to communicate with others about who we are and what we value. Now that I'm a healthy weight, I can walk into a store and know that if I see a shirt or dress that is cute, I can actually buy it—and it will be flattering on me. The freedom to express myself through my clothing is a completely new outlet.

- Now, if someone bumps into me and says, "Excuse me," it feels like they mean it, instead of meaning, "Get out of the way," which was how it felt before. I no longer feel like I'm on the defensive all the time. I can walk through a room or space without having to feel anxious from a purely logistical perspective. Before my weight loss, being in a space with a lot of people meant that I did not have the freedom to move about. It was not as simple as walking into another room when people were hanging around doorways and walkways, and I didn't know how to get through without making them physically step to the side. If a piece of furniture was too close to a wall or a table, I also didn't want people to judge me for trying to squeeze through or having to move it away so I could fit. It's been so much less stressful to simply be able to spatially maneuver within a place.

- I now get asked to sit in the middle seat of the car because I have the "smallest butt," instead of having to sit on the side while gripping on to the car handle to pull myself as far to the side as I could because I was worried that people would feel I was taking up too much room and making them uncomfortable.

- I have saved a lot of money that I used to spend on eating out or buying snacks. Since I just don't need as much food anymore, I get to save more. My food budget has dramatically reduced, even with the fresher, healthier foods that I buy. I've also learned to cook for myself, which has helped to reduce costs and given me the skillset to maneuver in the kitchen.

- My apartment and car are cleaner because I actually have the energy to get up and do something about a mess. I don't put off cleaning because it's no longer a physical chore, since I'm not carrying all that extra weight around with me; it's now just a regular chore. I am also not physically limited by what I can and can't clean—for example, I can actually reach around all the nooks and crannies to deep clean my bathroom and kitchen. I have the motivation to do these things because I get the reward of an organized and clean space, which has a mental benefit in return.

- I can sit on furniture and feel comfortable. I don't worry about whether or not other people can fit on the sofa with me or if I'm taking up so much space that maybe I should just stand instead. I used to opt for the floor when my feet hurt and would hug a pillow to cover my stomach—I don't do this anymore.
- When I get in the car, I can buckle a seatbelt without making the child safety lock go off or feel like I'm being strangled.
- My pants last so much longer because my thighs don't rub together and wear away the fabric.

Physical Changes

- I can see my collar bones for the first time in my life. They stick out! I think they're cute.
- I can see my feet when I look down, which takes my shoe obsession to a new level. Speaking of shoes, I went from a size 10.5/11 to a 9. This was honestly one of the most surprising parts of the weight loss. Shoes were always my favorite thing to buy in the past because, unlike clothes, they always fit. I had to get rid of so many shoes I loved once they were too big. But that meant I got to buy new shoes, which was a bonus.
- Now that I've lost weight, I can't see my stomach anymore because my breasts are in the way when I look down—which is a perspective I was not used to.

- I can't sleep on my side anymore without a pillow between my legs because my knees start to hurt when they are pressing on each other for too long.
- I have better posture and less stress on my back, which doesn't hurt me anymore.
- My feet and knees don't randomly hurt. In the past, I remember being in pain just from standing for too long. I couldn't walk for more than a mile without my feet feeling intense pain. People didn't understand how painful it really was and that I wasn't just being lazy; I legitimately had trouble keeping up because I was so uncomfortable. Now that I've lost 52 percent of my body weight, it's easy to see where that pain came from. At my heaviest, I was essentially carrying around another me!
- It now hurts my butt if I sit for too long. When I was heavier, it felt like I was going everywhere with a built-in pillow to sit on. Now that the extra fat is gone, sitting with my bone against a hard surface does get a little uncomfortable.
- Since I've become more active and involved in weight lifting, I have developed more muscle, on top of the killer calves I already had from carrying so much weight around. When I get lean enough, they are defined and even protrude a little bit. It's cool to see my hard work in the gym pay off in a visually rewarding way.

Health and Well-Being

- One of the greatest physical and mental health rewards that came with the weight loss is the ability to sleep through the whole night. I used to wake up a minimum of two times per night, but now I wake up well-rested, energized, and ready to start my day.

- My cholesterol levels have since gone down to normal levels. It was weird to go to the doctor and hear them say, "Everything's looking normal."
- I went from a hypertensive blood pressure (I had to wear a monitoring cuff for two days in eighth grade because my blood pressure was so high) to a normal blood pressure, with a resting heart rate of 52 beats per minute.
- I'm no longer anywhere close to being pre-diabetic.
- I don't feel bloated, crappy all the time, or sick from highly processed foods or sugar consumption. When I started eating less processed foods, I could actually feel a difference (even when I was obese!). It was powerful to see just how much I was affected by what I ate and the impact it had on my ability to do things.
- Going to the doctor is no longer a drag. In fact, I usually don't give it a second thought, and I find myself being more proactive about my health, such as scheduling checkups and vaccinations. In the past, my doctor used to only address my weight status instead of the reason I had come to see her. Now I feel like I can truly advocate for myself and my needs in a medical setting.
- Instead of worrying about what I look like or how my clothes fit or if I needed to readjust my clothes, I now have spare mental energy to dedicate to self-care and the other things I'm passionate about.
- I have gained so much knowledge about food and nutrition. Over the course of two years of losing weight, I read thousands of articles and books about food and nutrition. It seems that everyone has different opinions about the foods they think are best, but at least I know how to evaluate a nutrition label, what things to look for when I go grocery shopping, and

what substitutions to make when I want to make something a little healthier or more satiating. This knowledge is really empowering. It makes me feel like I have control over what I am putting in my body.

- I now take the stairs every single time out of habit. I like it because it's good exercise and also faster than the elevator most of the time, if you're traveling between just a few floors.

- I completed a half marathon (13.1 miles) without stopping! It was one of the most accomplished feelings I've ever experienced. Running, and exercising more generally, without all that extra weight is so much easier.

Honestly, I will say that all this is just the tip of the iceberg. Anyone who has lost a large amount of weight will also bring up different aspects of their lives that have changed. That's the beauty of all of this—it's all yours, and you get to find your way. I hope my sharing has showed you that you are not alone. You have allies you haven't met yet who will stand with you in solidarity. You have friends who will check in with you to see how you're doing. You also have yourself—and making peace with yourself is one of the most important things you'll do.

CHAPTER 27

A Gift to Yourself and a Gift to Others

Let your children be part of food
preparation and cooking. They'll learn
about following directions, measuring,
and cleaning up along the way

A Gift to Yourself

In the United States, more than a third of all adults are obese.[1] Why
is that? A large study showed that American adults gain an average of
almost a pound a year when they eat a typical Western diet, which is
high in convenient, processed foods. A pound a year may not sound
like much, but it adds up. In this study, those who gained the most
weight ate more potato chips, potatoes, sugar-sweetened drinks, processed meats, and red meat. Those who were the least likely to gain
weight ate a diet higher in vegetables, fruits, yogurt, whole grains, and
nuts. By the way, in this same study as well as in others, weight gain
was also associated with being less physically active, watching more
television, and not getting adequate sleep.[2] None of these findings
come as a surprise.

Also, not surprisingly, those who gain weight on unhealthy diets are the people at greatest risk for heart disease, obesity-related cancers, and other diseases and disabling conditions[3] that we've discussed before. On the other hand, if you're overweight and lose just 5 percent of your initial body weight and then maintain that weight loss for three years, you will reap the benefit of dramatically lowering your risk for those diseases[4]—as much as 50 percent for coronary heart disease and a 75 percent decrease for stroke.[5]

Many of the medical benefits of weight loss are directly related to the benefits of losing that weight through a healthy diet, as we discussed in Chapter 19. There are also some gifts specific to weight loss in women that we want to mention, which are related to the improved hormonal and reproductive function that comes with weight loss.

Improvement in symptoms associated with polycystic ovarian syndrome (PCOS)

Polycystic ovary syndrome (PCOS) is a hormonal disorder that affects at least 10 percent of women of reproductive age.[6] For most women, it begins in adolescence and generally includes irregular, heavy menstrual periods, signs of androgen excess (such as acne and excess facial hair), and obesity. Women who have PCOS are at increased risk of developing hypertension, type 2 diabetes, and cancer of the uterus. They may also have difficulty getting pregnant. While it is unclear what causes PCOS, it is very clear that weight loss helps.[7]

Fertility and pregnancy

Being at a healthy weight before and during pregnancy is good for both mother and baby. Not only is there a lower risk of pregnancy and delivery complications,[8] but a healthy weight is also associated with decreased risk for the baby to develop obesity, diabetes, and heart disease later in life.[9, 10]

Janice—I took the whole "eating for two" notion a little too seriously when I was pregnant. I remember repeating that mantra to myself when I was just a month or so pregnant, casually ignoring the fact that one of the two of us was the size of a lima bean. Pregnancy is most definitely not a time to try to lose weight, but it's a wonderful time to commit to healthy eating. It's the best baby gift ever!

Is "Fit and Fat" a Myth?

The answer to that question is: it's complicated. In a study of more than a hundred thousand men and women over a period of more than thirty years, overweight people with otherwise healthy lifestyles (meaning they exercised and didn't drink heavily or smoke) lived longer than overweight people without healthy habits. But they did not live as long as non-overweight people who also had healthy lifestyles.[11] Obese people are at increased risk for health problems, particularly cardiovascular disease, as well as earlier death, even if they are metabolically healthy.[12]

It's Never Too Late!

Here's the good news: many of these health problems are reversible!

- In a study of people age forty-five and older, those who adopted a healthy lifestyle (meaning at least five fruits and vegetables daily, regular exercise, and no tobacco) quickly lowered their risk for cardiovascular disease and earlier death.[13] They also changed their body contour by losing abdominal fat[14]—a nice bonus!
- In a study of people with obesity age sixty-five and older, there was increased physical fitness, strength, and balance in those

who changed to either a healthy weight-loss diet or an exercise program. The results were best for those who did both.[15]

- In a study of people with obesity age sixty and older who had mild cognitive impairment, weight loss was associated with improved cognition.[16]

A Gift to Your Family, Present and Future

Throughout this book, we hope we have convinced you that changing your relationship with food will reap fantastic physical and emotional rewards. Now, let's shift our focus to the rewards for your children.

Childhood obesity has been widely referred to as an "epidemic."[17] It has more than tripled in the past thirty years, and the Centers for Disease Control and Prevention has classified it as a "public health crisis." We don't need to tell you that overweight children have a tough time socially and medically.[18]

Children with obesity are more likely to suffer from depression and anxiety. They are more likely to be obese as adults.[19] They are more likely to develop early heart disease,[20] sleep disorders, breast cancer,[21] and joint problems.[22] They are more susceptible to developing type 2 diabetes at an early age—in fact, as early as age five.[23]

Janice—when I was in medical school, we didn't even call it "type 2 diabetes." Rather, the term we used was "adult-onset diabetes." We can't do that anymore because so many children now suffer from that disease.

The social consequences for children with obesity can be devastating. Overweight children (just like adults) suffer the cruel consequences of weight stigma, including being bullied, experiencing bias from teachers, and having fewer friends.[24]

Of course, for both children and adults, there are definitely genetic and metabolic predispositions that contribute to a greater likelihood of being overweight. But genetic tendency is *not* the same as destiny. You're aware as an adult of how difficult it is to change years-long habits and years-long shame. Getting your kids on a healthy road is one of the greatest gifts you can give them.

Now, let's return to the age-old assumption that food equals love. Food is used to express affection, to comfort and console, to bribe—you name it. An iconic photograph of someone who is a "great mom" typically shows her in the kitchen, in an apron, removing a pan of home-baked cookies from the oven, ready to serve them to her children who sit adoringly at the table in happy anticipation. But let's face it: the way many of us feed our children, and the way food corporations *encourage* us to feed our children, puts them on a trajectory of potential misery. Luckily, if you're a parent or caretaker, you are now in a wonderful position to dramatically shift this trajectory.

The most effective treatment for overweight and obese children and adolescents is, not surprisingly, a combination of changes in diet and exercise.[25] By feeding your children in a healthy way and by encouraging them to be physically active, you will have a dramatic impact on not just their current physical and emotional well-being but also their future health and vitality. This regimen is much more likely to succeed when the eating and activity changes are incorporated into the entire family's habits.[26] In other words, the positive changes you make for yourself will reinforce those same changes in your kids.

Jae—*I didn't grow up eating healthy foods in a healthy way, but now I have the chance to change my future family's course. I want to set an example for my siblings. I want to show my future nieces and nephews that I take care of and respect my body for the things it lets me do. I want to show them that by giving them healthy foods, I'm respecting and caring for their bodies, too. That's a real gift.*

Janice—I love that I can go on walks with my children, and I want to stay healthy so I can continue to do this with them and, if I'm lucky, with their children for a long time to come. I'm proud to do everything I can to prevent me from being dependent on them when I'm older.

It may feel like society is conspiring against you when you try to make these changes for your family. There is a constant barrage of advertising aimed at children and enticing them with sweet and processed foods and drinks. School lunches are not helping the situation either[27] (and we strongly support any efforts you can make to encourage your schools to make substantive changes in their food offerings). However, note that children's preferences for fatty and sugary foods and drinks "are already determined by the time they enter school."[28]

You Can Stop the Fat-Shaming Cycle!

Here's the biggest gift you can give to your kids: make a decision to talk to them about food in a way that stresses health and is never shaming. As we discussed in Chapter 24, shame and guilt will not motivate you, and they will not motivate children, either. Shame is destructive at every age. You probably already know all too well how it has affected you. In fact, the biggest gift you can give to your kids is to be less critical of *yourself*. The way you treat yourself serves as a model for your children.

Janice—The majority of my patients who experienced weight-associated shame told me that not only did the shame began in childhood, and not only was the shame most related to comments made by a parent, but my patients could also still remember the exact words their parents used—and those words still burned. Here are some of the things that were said to them:

"You need to go on a diet."
"Do you really want to eat that?"
"I'll buy you new clothes if you lose weight."
"This dessert is not for you."
"Boys don't like fat girls."

A few suggestions:

- Make healthy eating and exercise habits a family affair. Model the changes you wish to see in your kids. Don't have soda or sugar-packed cereal in the house. Pack carrot sticks and almonds instead of chips in their lunches. Have contests at dinner to see who can eat the most colorful foods. Your own journey is a great opportunity to stop the cycle of shaming children about their appearance.

- Were you encouraged (or forced) to be a member of the "Clean Plate Club"? We think that's a tradition that should end right now. Think about it: you force children to eat more than they want to in order to "reward" them with dessert. Dinner, which should be a happy time of sharing, turns into an ordeal for everyone involved.

- Using smaller plates, as we mentioned in Chapter 22, tricks your brain and your stomach into thinking you have more food on the plate. This is certainly true for children as well. We recommend smaller plates, bowls, glasses—and even spoons! All have been shown to be effective.[29]

- Get your kids involved with food shopping and preparation. For example, if they're old enough, let them help make the shopping list. Offer them choices—of course, not a choice between broccoli and M&M's, but maybe between broccoli and asparagus. When they're at the grocery store with you, teach them how to read labels and work with a budget. When you get home, let your children be part of food preparation and cooking. They'll learn about following directions, measuring, and cleaning up along the way. When your kids have participated in making food, they'll be both curious and proud to eat it.

While two-thirds of children with obesity go on to be obese adults, let's focus on the one-third who lose weight and who do *not* become obese. How do they accomplish that? Here's what they have in common when they become adolescents who "exit obesity":[30]

- They eat less fast food
- They reduce their "screen time"
- They eat more fruits and vegetables
- They're more physically active
- They partake in a higher number of family meals

Let us be clear: you may not be able to control a world of cruel people, fast food, and consequences of technology that have led us to become a more sedentary society. But you *do* have influence over your children regarding having healthy foods in the home and encouraging more physical activity and less screen time for the family. Most of all, you can make your home a shame-free zone.

Conclusion

Here's our final message.

Jae—*Sharing the story about my significant weight loss in this book was incredibly difficult for me. Sometimes, I was downright resistant. Sometimes, my amazing coauthor had to wait patiently as I worked through my own personal struggles to put very painful memories and strong emotions into words on paper. I've shared personal moments in this book that I don't even talk to my friends about, and I'll be honest, it scares me. I am not usually so open with my life and the times when I felt like I wasn't worth much.*

I do not like talking about my weight loss, but this is not because I'm ashamed of who I was, but rather because it is not how I define myself. I am so much more—I have done a lot of things in my academic life and have so many friendships that I value deeply—all of which are not part of my weight loss.

Janice wasn't kidding when she recounted our first meeting together. I really didn't think that what I had done was a big deal. But in writing this book and talking about my own experiences with Janice, I've realized that losing more than half my body weight is not something to be taken lightly. There are millions of people out there who are in the same shoes as I was and who just need to know that making sustainable, lasting change is not out of reach. It's not mythical, it's not just for some people. It's for everyone.

If telling my story can inspire just one person, then this was all worth it.

Janice—*I have instructed my children that when I'm on my deathbed, they are to bring me a bacon cheeseburger, followed by a hot fudge sundae. In a perverse way, I look forward to that. But until that time, I'll continue to eat and move in a way that will, hopefully, allow me to be hauling compost in my garden during the afternoon before I settle into that deathbed and await my last supper. That's my hope for myself.*

In the book Gorge,[1] *Kara Richardson Whitely's memoir of climbing Mt. Kilimanjaro when she weighed three hundred pounds, she describes how one night, when all the climbers were in their tents, she heard several of the guides laughing derisively about her. The next day, she insisted that Kenedy, the guide with whom she had been climbing, tell her what was going on. He told her that the other guides didn't think she'd make it to the top. "Did you make any money bets?" she asked. "You should," she said, pausing. "Bet on me. Bet on me."*

Jae and I placed bets on ourselves, that we could—and deserved to— make big changes in our lives. Bet on yourself, too. That's our hope for you.

APPENDIX

Selected Recipes

We've created a rather eclectic collection of recipes, each one for a specific reason that we'll explain. You'll notice that most of these offerings are plant-based, with a few fish and seafood recipes tossed in. Our goal is to offer you suggestions for delicious foods that may expand your cooking horizons and make your body happy. Enjoy!

VEGETABLES

J&J's Roasted Summer Vegetables

Serves 8—or 1 or 2 people for several days

As you know by now, the key to our sustained weight loss, and not to mention good health, can be summed up in one word: vegetables. When we talk about vegetables, we're not referring to starchier vegetables such as potatoes and corn. If weight loss is a goal for you and you're not eating a lot of vegetables, you simply will not be able to eat enough without feeling deprived. Whenever possible, buy seasonal, local vegetables.

Why do we love this recipe? When we come home from work or school, tired and hungry, we need something in the refrigerator that we can eat *right now*. Roasted vegetables fill that bill, either cold or reheated. We know ourselves: if there's nothing satisfying and healthy to eat available, we're going to find that lost stash of peanut butter crackers, rationalize why we "deserve" to eat them after a hard day, and then, well, you know the rest.

You can make this recipe with all kinds of variations: add chopped fresh tomatoes or canned tomatoes, or add or substitute any other vegetables you like, such as fennel, asparagus, broccoli, and Brussels sprouts. You can make this a full meal by adding a protein, such as chick peas or cooked shrimp, or by using this as a filling for an omelet.

Ingredients
4 small eggplants (about 2 pounds), cut into 1-inch pieces*
4 small zucchinis (about 2 pounds), cut into 1-inch pieces
3 medium red bell peppers, cut into 1-inch pieces
3 medium onions, peeled and cut into 1-inch chunks

3 peeled garlic cloves, whole (to mash later) or minced

2 tablespoons extra-virgin olive oil

1 tablespoon chopped fresh thyme (or 1 teaspoon dried)

1–4 tablespoons chopped fresh rosemary (or 1 teaspoon dried)

1 tablespoon chopped fresh basil (don't bother with dried if you don't have fresh)

1 tablespoon red wine vinegar or balsamic vinegar (optional)

Preparation

1. Preheat oven to 375°F.
2. Line two rimmed baking sheets with foil.
3. Toss eggplant, zucchini, peppers, onions, garlic, and oil together in a large bowl. Divide evenly between prepared baking sheets, spreading out the vegetables in a single layer.
4. Roast, stirring once, until vegetables are the tenderness you like, 30 to 60 minutes. Ideally, rotate the baking sheets halfway through roasting time.
5. When the vegetables are done, add the thyme, rosemary, and basil. If you like, add the vinegar. If you used whole roasted garlic, mash and add to the vegetables, and stir.

Note

*We prefer small varieties of eggplant—Italian or Japanese—because they're less bitter and don't require salting, rinsing, drying, and otherwise making you want to give up on eggplant altogether.

Joanna's Cauliflower Quinoa Puttanesca

Serves 4

Janice—*My daughter Joanna is not only a brilliant classics professor who looks like the Mona Lisa; she is also a fabulous cook. Here's one of her recipes and the reasons why I love it: 1. I love Joanna and all things related to her. 2. I love saying "puttanesca," which is a melodious and charming word (and which means prostitute, apparently).*

The dish is easy, beautiful, and full of flavor. You can make some of it or all ahead of time. Quinoa, a high-protein healthy grain, really shines here. Also, you can make the dish even heartier by adding white beans, cooked shrimp, shredded cooked chicken, or other proteins.

Ingredients

1 head cauliflower, pulled apart into florets
1 tablespoon extra-virgin olive oil
1–2 cloves garlic, minced or smashed or whole
2–3 anchovy fillets
½ teaspoon red pepper flakes (optional)
1 cup quinoa
1 (14.5-oz) can diced tomatoes, drained
10 pitted Kalamata olives
1 tablespoon capers
Chopped parsley or cilantro

Preparation

1. Preheat oven to 350°F.
2. Place cauliflower florets in a foil-lined baking sheet.
3. Combine the oil, garlic, anchovies, and red pepper flakes in a small bowl, and then toss with the cauliflower.

4. Bake until the florets are the desired tenderness, around 15 minutes.
5. In the meantime, cook the quinoa according to package directions.
6. Place the cooked quinoa in a bowl, and top with the cauliflower mixture, tomatoes, olives, and capers. Sprinkle chopped parsley or cilantro over the top.

"Umami Bomb" Roasted Portabella Mushrooms

Serves 2–4

Janice—*My mother was the best cook I've ever known. Really. The chicken soup she made for the holidays was legendary. There was a problem, though. Every time I had that soup, I would get a raging headache, my face would turn bright red, and my jaw would tighten. I didn't correlate this with her "secret" ingredient, monosodium glutamate (MSG), a flavor enhancer that causes those symptoms in some people. I thought my troubles were caused by the stress of a holiday with a slightly crazy family, but now I know better. I mean, my family is, indeed, slightly crazy, but it was the MSG that was the problem.*

MSG is a potent member of a group of chemicals called glutamates that give certain foods the property known as *umami*. Along with sweet, sour, bitter, and salty, umami is a taste category perhaps best described as savory. It adds an incredible amount of flavor. What's more, umami increases the sense of fullness and decreases the desire for added salt. The good news is that there are many umami-rich foods that contain glutamates that are not MSG and that do not usually cause MSG-associated problems. Seaweed, mushrooms, Parmesan cheese, and fermented foods such as miso and soy products are particularly rich in umami. Other umami-rich foods include tomatoes, balsamic vinegar, cured meats (the reason we all love bacon so much, alas), shellfish, and anchovies. For several of these foods, notably tomatoes and mushrooms, cooking them increases the umami effect. Be aware, though, that sometimes even these non-MSG umami foods are "trigger foods" for people with migraine headaches.

Combining umami-rich foods exponentially increases their intensity, resulting in what has been called "umami bombs." Here's a recipe for one of our favorites.

Ingredients

1 tablespoon olive oil

2 tablespoons dark soy sauce

2 tablespoons balsamic or red wine vinegar

1–2 cloves garlic, minced

1–2 teaspoons miso (any color you like)

1 teaspoon fish sauce (optional)

Italian parsley, minced

2 large portabella mushrooms, stems removed

1–2 teaspoons Parmesan cheese, freshly grated (optional)

Preparation

1. Preheat oven to 400°F.
2. In a baking dish, mix the olive oil, soy sauce, vinegar, garlic, miso, fish sauce, and parsley.
3. Wipe the mushrooms clean with a damp paper towel.
4. Place mushroom caps upside down in the marinade, and spoon the marinade into the cups. Marinate for 15 to 60 minutes.
5. Transfer the dish to the preheated oven. Bake for 20 to 30 minutes until the mushrooms are soft, flipping the mushrooms about halfway through.* Before removing from the oven, sprinkle on the Parmesan, and bake another minute or so.

Serving Options

Serve the mushrooms with the sauce over steamed kale, spinach, or Swiss chard. Cut up the cooked mushrooms and mix them with grains or rice or in a salad.

Note

*If you prefer, instead of roasting the mushrooms, you can grill them after they're marinated. Grill over medium-low heat for 5 minutes on each side, or until the mushrooms are soft.

Caramelized Sweet Potatoes, Two Ways

Serves 4

Here's why we love sweet potatoes (as compared to regular potatoes): for one thing, they're sweet! It may surprise you, then, to learn that sweet potatoes have a lower glycemic index than white potatoes. In other words, they raise blood sugar levels less. Sweet potatoes also have fewer calories and way more vitamin A than white potatoes. Plus, they're just so pretty.

Ingredients
4 sweet potatoes
1–2 tablespoons extra-virgin olive oil
Salt and pepper (seasoning choice #1)
Cinnamon and pinch of cayenne pepper (seasoning choice #2)

Preparation
1. Scrub sweet potatoes and dry them. Slice on the bias (so there's more surface area) into ½-inch or so slices. Place in a foil-lined baking pan.
2. Combine the olive oil with seasoning choice #1 or #2 in a small bowl.*
3. Brush the potato slices with the oil mixture. Turn slices over and brush again.
4. Place in a cold oven and then bake at 450°F for 10 minutes.**
5. Flip the slices and bake for 5 or 10 minutes or more until fork-tender.

Note

*We like the version with seasoning #1 to accompany savory foods and the version with seasoning #2 as a dessert.

**Why the cold oven to start? By putting the potatoes in a cold oven, that allows for greater caramelization to occur. Joanna taught us this. Brilliant!

SOUPS

Roasted Vegetable and Bean Soup

Serves 8

Vegetable soup can be so boring if the vegetables are pale, mushy, and bland. Not this recipe! Roasting the vegetables first makes them so much more flavorful, and the beans add a wallop of filling, nutrient-rich, protein-packed fiber. You can also make this with fall and root vegetables, such as sweet potatoes, beets, parsnips, and butternut squash. This soup freezes well.

Ingredients
1 large or 2–3 small eggplants, cut into 1-inch chunks
2 zucchini, cut into 1-inch chunks
2 red bell peppers, cut into 1-inch chunks
½ pound fresh mushrooms, preferably cremini or shitake, quartered
1–2 sweet potatoes, peeled and cut into 1-inch chunks
1 leek, white part only, sliced
8 garlic cloves, whole and unpeeled
2 tablespoons extra-virgin olive oil, divided
8 cups vegetable or chicken broth
1 tablespoon balsamic or red wine vinegar
1 (15-oz) can white beans (cannellini or great northern)*
1 (15-oz) can kidney beans, rinsed and drained*
1 (15-oz) can garbanzo beans (chickpeas), rinsed and drained*
1 teaspoon dried thyme
1 teaspoon dried rosemary, crushed

Salt and pepper
Parmesan cheese, freshly grated (optional)

Preparation

1. Line two large baking pans with foil.
2. Place eggplant, zucchini, peppers, mushrooms, potato, leek, and garlic in the pans.
3. Toss each pan of vegetables with 1 tablespoon oil each, or just enough to coat them lightly.
4. Place the pans in a cold oven. Turn on oven to 425°F. Bake for 15 minutes and then switch the positions of the pans if they're on two racks. Bake for another 15 to 30 minutes, until the vegetables are just softened.
5. In a large pot, add the broth, vinegar, beans, and seasonings.
6. Cut off one end of each garlic clove, remove the skin, and squeeze out the pulp into the pot. Add the roasted vegetables. Bring to a boil, and then immediately reduce the heat.
7. Cover and simmer for 10 minutes or until just heated through. If you like, top each serving with a bit of grated Parmesan.

Note

*Dried beans are cheaper than canned beans, and some people think they're more flavorful. Feel free to use dried beans that you have soaked and cooked instead of canned ones. We just usually can't seem to remember to do that ahead of time.

Mushroom Farro Soup

Serves 6

This recipe is adapted from Deb Perelman's website, Smitten Kitchen. Deb is one of the best writers and cooks we know of. This recipe is flavorful and nutrient-packed; it also freezes well. Farro is an ancient grain that has a lovely chewiness to it. Substitute barley if you like.

***Janice**—I like to add thinly sliced fresh spinach to each bowl when I serve this. Don't add it to the pot ahead of time, though, or the spinach will get mushy.*

Ingredients
⅓ cup dried porcini mushrooms
1 onion
1 carrot
2 cloves garlic, peeled
1 pound fresh mushrooms, preferably cremini or shitake, cleaned and trimmed
2 tablespoons extra-virgin olive oil
½ cup farro or barley
6 cups vegetable, mushroom, or chicken stock
¼ cup dry sherry
1 tablespoon tomato paste
1 tablespoon miso, dissolved in a little hot water or stock
Salt and pepper to taste
1 tablespoon balsamic or sherry vinegar

Preparation
1. Cover dried mushrooms with 1 cup boiling water, and set aside for 20 minutes.

2. In the meantime, start chopping the vegetables. If you want to do this by hand, dice the carrot and onion so they are nice and even, and then mince the garlic and slice the fresh mushrooms. If you want to make your life easier, cut the carrot and onion into big chunks and pulse them in a food processor until they're chopped into little pieces. Remove and set aside; then, with the motor still running, throw the garlic into the processor and let it process for several seconds. Remove the garlic, set aside, and add the fresh mushrooms and pulse until they're the size you like.

3. Heat oil in large pot. Sauté onions and carrots over medium-low heat until onions begin to turn golden, about 10 minutes. Add the garlic, and sauté for 30 seconds. Add the mushrooms, and cook until they begin to release their liquid, about 5 to 10 minutes. Raise the heat to medium-high, and add the farro or barley. Sauté it for 1 minute or so, and then add the broth, sherry, and tomato paste.

4. Strain the porcinis, and save the water. Chop the porcinis by hand or in the food processor. Add to the pot. Stir the miso into the mushroom liquid, and add to the pot. Season with salt and pepper, and simmer for about 40 minutes, until grains are tender. Stir in the vinegar.

Sweet & Sour Cabbage Soup

Serves 4

Yes, this recipe includes a bit of brown sugar, but that ingredient makes all the difference. Feel free to try honey if you prefer. This soup freezes well.

Janice—*With this recipe, I'm channeling my mother, whose cabbage soup was legendary. Forgive me, Mom—no fatty meat or dollop of sour cream in this version.*

Ingredients

1 tablespoon canola oil

1 onion, halved and sliced

½ head thinly sliced green cabbage (about 6 cups)

1 (14.5-oz) can diced tomatoes

1 teaspoon caraway seeds (optional)

4 cups beef stock or water

2–4 tablespoons cider vinegar

1–3 teaspoons fresh lemon juice

1–3 tablespoons brown sugar

½ teaspoon smoked paprika

¼ cup raisins (optional)

Salt and pepper to taste

Preparation

1. Heat oil in a pot over medium heat. Add the onion, cabbage, and tomatoes. Cook until the cabbage is soft, 5 to 10 minutes.
2. Add the caraway seeds, stock, vinegar, lemon juice, sugar, and paprika. If you like, add raisins. Stir.
3. Cover and simmer over medium heat for 15 minutes.
4. Season with salt and pepper to taste.

SALADS

Kale and Beet Salad with Goat Cheese

Serves 4

Even if Christmas food may seem to be all about the cookies, at some point, even we cookie lovers need to change it up a bit. This red and green salad is delicious, refreshing, and drop-dead gorgeous, never mind healthy, on a Christmas dinner table or during any other time of the year. While we can't locate his exact recipe, we're pretty sure the inspiration came from the fabulous Israeli chef Yotam Ottolenghi.

Ingredients
4 beets, peeled and cut into chunks
2 tablespoons extra-virgin olive oil
1 bunch kale, thick central vein removed, torn into pieces*

VINAIGRETTE DRESSING**
2 tablespoons extra-virgin olive oil
2 teaspoons balsamic or red wine vinegar
2 oranges, peeled and cut into slices
2–4 tablespoons toasted pecans, walnuts, or pistachios
2–4 tablespoons crumbled goat cheese
Pomegranate seeds

Preparation
1. Toss the beets with the 2 tablespoons of olive oil and bake at 425°F until fork-tender. The length of time will depend on the size of your chunks. Check every 10 minutes or so.
2. Place the kale on a platter or in a bowl.

3. Mix the vinaigrette ingredients and toss with the kale.
4. Then top with everything else, with the pomegranate seeds on top, so they look like sparkly jewels!

Note

*We prefer the flatter types of kale, such as lacinato or dinosaur, but feel free to use curly, if you prefer.

**You can make a vinaigrette dressing with two-thirds olive oil and one-third balsamic vinegar or lemon juice.

Szechuan Cucumber Salad

Serves 2–4

There are many versions of this flavorful, refreshing recipe; but we think this one is the best.

Ingredients

¼ cup chopped peanuts

1 tablespoon sesame seeds

½ cup rice vinegar

1 tablespoon tamari or soy sauce

1 teaspoon sesame oil

½ serrano or jalapeno pepper, minced

1–2 teaspoons minced fresh ginger

2 cucumbers

1 small red onion, very thinly sliced

1 tablespoon chopped cilantro

Preparation

1. In a dry pan over medium heat, cook the peanuts and sesame seeds, stirring constantly for 1 minute. Set aside.
2. Whisk together vinegar, tamari or soy sauce, sesame oil, pepper, and ginger.
3. Halve cucumbers lengthwise, seed, and thinly slice crosswise.*
4. Place the cucumbers and onions in a bowl. Pour dressing over, and stir. Refrigerate for 1 to 2 hours.
5. When ready to serve, garnish with cilantro, peanuts, and sesame seeds.

Note

*A serrated spoon, sometimes called a grapefruit spoon, makes easy work of seeding cucumbers (and melons, winter squashes, etc.). Better yet, if you use English cucumbers, you won't have to deal with any seeds at all.

Curried Lentil Salad

Serves 6–8

This recipe is unusual and delicious. It's good in both the summer and winter, and it lasts in the refrigerator for days and days (if there's any left)!

Ingredients

CURRIED VINAIGRETTE
⅔ cup extra-virgin olive oil
¼ cup balsamic or red wine vinegar
1–3 teaspoons curry powder

SALAD
1 pound red lentils (a little more than 2 cups)
1 large onion, finely chopped
1 cup currants
½ cup capers, drained
¼ cup chopped scallions, for garnish (optional)

Preparation

1. Combine all the curried vinaigrette ingredients, and set aside.
2. Wash the lentils, and cook them in a pot of boiling water for 5 minutes, or until just tender. Drain, rinse, and place in a large bowl.
3. Pour in the vinaigrette, and combine.
4. Add the onion, currants, and capers. Stir well. Let marinate at least overnight.
5. If you like, garnish with scallions.

BEANS & GRAINS

Vegetarian Chili

Serves 4–6

This version of chili is delicious, healthy, and serves a big crowd. It also freezes well. The eggplant adds a nice meatiness.

Ingredients
1 eggplant
½ cup extra-virgin olive oil, divided
2 cloves garlic, peeled
½ jalapeño pepper, seeded
1 stalk celery, cut into large chunks
2 onions, peeled and cut into large chunks
1 green or red bell pepper, seeded and cut into large chunks
3 carrots, peeled and cut into large chunks
½ pound mushrooms, cleaned and trimmed
2 tablespoons chili powder
1 tablespoon ground cumin
1 teaspoon dried basil
1 teaspoon dried oregano
¼ teaspoon red pepper flakes
Salt and pepper to taste
1 cup tomato juice
1 cup bulgur wheat
1 (28-oz) can diced tomatoes
2 (14-oz) cans kidney beans, drained

Continued on next page

2 tablespoons fresh lemon juice

3 tablespoons tomato paste

1 tablespoon Worcestershire sauce

¼ cup red or white wine

2 tablespoons chopped canned green chilies

Preparation

1. Preheat oven to 350°F.
2. Slice the eggplant into ½- to 1-inch slices, and cut the slices into chunks. Place in a bowl.
3. Pour 1 to 2 tablespoons of the oil into the bowl and toss with the eggplant.
4. Transfer the eggplant to a baking pan in a single layer, and bake for 3 minutes. Turn the slices over, and bake for another 3 minutes. Set aside.
5. If you prefer to work by hand, mince the garlic and jalapeño, then finely chop the celery, onions, bell pepper, and carrots. If you prefer to use a food processor, pulse the garlic and jalapeño first, and then chop the celery, onions, bell pepper, and carrots into chunks.
6. In a large pot, heat the rest of the olive oil over medium heat. Add the chopped garlic, jalapeño, celery, onions, bell pepper, and carrots, as well as all the spices. Stir and cook for 2 minutes.
7. Add the eggplant and the remaining ingredients. Bring to a boil, stirring. Reduce the heat and simmer for 20 minutes, uncovered. If you want to thin out the chili a bit, add more tomato juice.

Black Bean Burgers

Serves 4

We played around with a lot of recipes, and we swear this is the best black bean burger in the whole wide world!

Ingredients
1–2 cloves garlic, peeled
2 medium portabella mushrooms, cleaned
1 medium onion
½ green pepper
4 tablespoons canola oil, divided
1 egg, beaten
2 tablespoons Dijon mustard
1–2 tablespoons maple syrup
1–2 tablespoons Worcestershire sauce
½ cup stale bread crumbs, preferably whole-grain
1 (15-oz) can black beans, rinsed and well-drained

Preparation
1. Mince the garlic, and coarsely chop the mushrooms, onion, and pepper. If you prefer, process the garlic in the food processor, and then add the mushrooms, onion, and pepper. Pulse until you have a coarse chop.
2. Heat 2 tablespoons of oil over low-medium heat. Add garlic, onions, mushrooms, and pepper. Cook for a few minutes, until softened. Turn off the heat, and let the mixture cool a bit.
3. Combine the egg, mustard, syrup, and Worcestershire sauce in a large bowl. Add the bread crumbs, and mash until well mixed.

4. Place the cooked vegetable mixture and the black beans in a food processor. Pulse a few times until the pieces are small. Don't overdo it, though—you don't want a smooth, gluey paste.

5. Add the black bean mixture to the egg mixture and combine well. Shape into patties as best you can.

6. Wipe out the pan you used before, and heat the remaining 2 tablespoons of oil over medium heat. Place the patties in the pan, and leave them alone, letting them cook for 7 minutes. This is your best chance for them to form a bit of a crust and hold together well. Then carefully flip them over and cook for another 7 minutes. Voila!

Note

This recipe makes around 4 patties, but you may want to double it and freeze some.

White Beans with Grilled Broccoli and Parmesan

Serves 4

Parmesan cheese offers a lot of umami flavor—a bang for your calorie and health buck. A tablespoon of grated Parmesan has only 22 calories. If you throw a Parmesan rind into the pot while you're making soup with vegetables or beans, you'll be thrilled with the results. What's more, most lactose-intolerant people have no problem with aged Parmesan (and other aged cheeses). This recipe is terrific with cooked shrimp.

Ingredients
1 bunch broccoli
3 tablespoons extra-virgin olive oil, divided
1 clove garlic, minced
1 lemon
2 (15-oz) cans cannellini or great northern beans, drained and
    rinsed (or use cooked dried beans)
5 ounces or so (1 bag) arugula
1 can anchovies (optional)
3 or 4 strips of Parmesan cheese

Preparation
1. Cut the broccoli in florets. Rinse and drain.
2. Steam or microwave the florets for 1 to 2 minutes, until not quite cooked. Drain.
3. Combine 1 tablespoon of oil with the minced garlic, and pour over the broccoli.
4. Grill the broccoli over medium heat for 1 minute on each side or until you think it's done. Alternatively, you can roast the florets in a 425°F preheated oven for 10 minutes or so.

5. Peel some strips of lemon peel, and then juice half of the lemon, or enough to get 1 tablespoon of juice. If you like, slice the other lemon half to use as a garnish.

6. Combine the lemon juice with the remaining 2 tablespoons of olive oil.

7. Arrange the beans, arugula, and broccoli on a platter. Place the anchovies and Parmesan strips over the top. Drizzle the lemon-juice-and-olive-oil mixture over everything. Place the anchovies and Parmesan strips over the top.

Savory Breakfast, Lunch, or Dinner Bowl

Serves 4

Jae—*Preparing dinner bowls with other people can be a great way to cook with friends or family. When I'm with Janice, one of our go-to dinners is a large bowl of filling and varied ingredients. I love eating this way because we get to spend time preparing a meal together, while at the same time customizing our own bowls. I like using bell pepper, tomato, or portabella mushroom cap for my ingredients.*

By the way, a bowl doesn't have to be an actual bowl. A big plate works, too!

Ingredients

1 bunch kale, stemmed and chopped
Salt and pepper to taste
2 tablespoons extra-virgin olive oil + 1 tablespoon, if necessary
1 onion, chopped
2 tomatoes, chopped
Other vegetables of your choice, such as zucchini, bell peppers, broccoli, and/or mushrooms, chopped
1 clove garlic, minced
3 cups cooked quinoa* or other grain
4 eggs or 1 pound firm or extra firm tofu, dried and cut into cubes
2 avocadoes, halved, pitted, skinned, and sliced
Hummus or plain Greek yogurt
Chopped nuts and/or seeds (optional)

Preparation

1. Place skillet over medium-high heat. Add kale and 3 tablespoons of water. Cover and cook, stirring once, until wilted, 2 to 3 minutes. Season with salt and pepper; transfer to plate.

2. Heat 2 tablespoons of oil in the pan over low-medium heat, and add the onion. Add the tomatoes and other vegetables of your choice. Cook, stirring frequently, a few minutes, until softened. Add the garlic, and stir another 30 seconds. Stir in quinoa, and heat through. Season with more salt and pepper. Remove to bowls, placing the vegetables on top of the quinoa.

3. Cook the eggs however you like: scrambled or fried in the pan you've already used, or poached or boiled. If using tofu, heat 1 tablespoon of oil at medium heat, add the tofu, and cook at medium heat for 5 to 8 minutes.**

4. Place the eggs or tofu on top of the bowls, then place the avocado slices. Finally, top with hummus or yogurt and, if you like, the nuts and seeds.

Note

*Quinoa tastes nuttier (and, in our opinion, better) if you first cook it in a dry saucepan for a few minutes until it darkens a bit in color. Then, add the water and cook as usual. An added bonus if you use this method is that you don't have to bother rinsing the quinoa first. **If you're using tofu and want to add a little kick, add 1 teaspoon of curry powder to the oil or 1 tablespoon of soy sauce when you cook the tofu.

For this recipe, feel free to prepare quinoa and vegetables the night before and simply store in the refrigerator.

FISH & SEAFOOD

Mustard & Maple-Glazed Stuffed Salmon

Serves 6

This recipe is easy, healthy, gorgeous, and perfect for company. You can play with the stuffing ingredients if you wish. We've chosen the vegetables based on personal preference, color, and texture, but you may prefer to omit some or add others.

Ingredients
1 tablespoon extra-virgin olive oil

VEGETABLES FOR STUFFING, SUCH AS:
½ red pepper, chopped or thinly sliced
½ onion, chopped or thinly sliced
1 cup mushrooms, chopped or thinly sliced
1 large handful fresh baby spinach or frozen spinach, thawed and dried
½ cup pine nuts, toasted (optional)
1 pound salmon filet, butterflied (i.e., cut in half horizontally almost all the way through, so it opens like a book)

GLAZE
1 tablespoon Dijon mustard
1 teaspoon maple syrup or honey
1 tablespoon soy sauce or tamari

Preparation
1. Preheat oven to 350°F.

2. Heat the oil on low-medium heat and sauté the vegetables except the spinach for a few minutes until they are softened. Turn off the heat and stir in the spinach. Place the vegetables (and nuts, if you're using them) between the two salmon layers.
3. Combine the glaze ingredients in a small bowl. Brush the glaze over the top of the salmon.
4. Place the salmon on a foil-lined baking sheet.* Place in oven and bake for 30 minutes.

Note

*The foil is *not* optional if you ever want to be able to use that pan again!

Baked Cod with Provençale Sauce

Serves 4

Cod is a healthy, mild-tasting flaky fish. Pacific (as opposed to Atlantic) cod is abundant. It can be baked, broiled, poached, or sautéed. You can use it in soups or fish tacos. On its own, though, it can be a little boring, which is why we use it with this Provençale sauce. We think you'll agree that the sauce makes this fish become so good.

Ingredients
1 tablespoon extra-virgin olive oil
1 onion, chopped or halved and thinly sliced
1 green, red, or yellow bell pepper, seeded and chopped or sliced
    into strips
1 tablespoon chopped fresh thyme or 2 teaspoons dried
½ teaspoon fennel seeds
2 anchovies, minced (optional)
2–3 cloves garlic, minced
1 (14.5-oz) can diced tomatoes in juice
12 Kalamata or Niçoise olives
½ cup dry white wine
2 tablespoons tomato paste
1 tablespoon capers, drained
4 (4–6-oz) pieces cod or other white meat fish
1 teaspoon extra-virgin olive oil
½ cup fresh basil, chopped (optional)

Preparation
1. Preheat oven to 400°F.

2. To make the sauce, heat 1 tablespoon of oil in a large skillet over medium heat. Add onion, bell peppers, thyme, and fennel seeds to the skillet. If you like, add anchovies. Sauté until onion softens, about 5 minutes. Add garlic and cook another 30 seconds. Add tomatoes with juice, olives, wine, tomato paste, and capers. Bring to a boil. Reduce heat to medium-low, cover, and simmer for 10 minutes.

3. Put half of sauce in a large glass baking dish.

4. Pat the cod dry with paper towels. Place cod in the baking dish on top of the sauce. Brush the cod with 1 teaspoon of olive oil.

5. Cover the dish with a piece of aluminum foil, and bake for 10 minutes. Spoon the other half of the sauce over the cod, and bake another 15 minutes, uncovered.

6. If you like, add the basil over the top of the sauce.

Scallops with Orange, Spinach & Cucumber

Serves 4

Janice—*I once attended a lecture by Drew Ramsey, a psychiatrist, farmer, and cookbook author; and I was impressed by the depth of his knowledge of nutrition. This is an adaptation of one of his recipes in his book* Eat Complete.[2]

Ingredients

2 cucumbers, thinly sliced

3 tablespoons rice or apple cider vinegar, divided

¼ teaspoon salt

2 oranges

2 tablespoons extra-virgin olive oil, divided

¼ teaspoon ground pepper

¼ teaspoon paprika

16 sea scallops

4 big handfuls baby spinach

Preparation

1. Combine the cucumbers, 2 tablespoons of vinegar, and salt in a bowl. Set aside.

2. Grate the peel from the oranges, and place the zest in a small bowl along with 1 tablespoon of oil and the remaining 1 tablespoon of vinegar. Set aside.

3. Cut each orange into ½-inch slices and then cut each slice into quarters. Set aside.

4. Combine pepper and paprika in a shallow dish. Place scallops in the spice mixture and turn over to cover both sides.

5. Heat the remaining 1 tablespoon of oil in a large pan over medium-high heat. Cook the scallops in a single layer, turning once, for a total of 4 minutes, or until the scallops are no longer translucent in the center.

6. Divide the spinach on 4 plates. Top with scallops, cucumbers, and orange sections.

Shrimp with Pesto Zucchini "Noodles"

Serves 4

Vegetable "noodles" are all the rage, and for good reason. They're delicious and fun, especially for kids. If you haven't used a spiralizer, try it—the basic ones are cheap and work well enough.

Yes, homemade pesto is best, but store-bought or premade pesto is great, too. Pesto is easy to keep on hand in the freezer. You can also keep a bag of frozen uncooked shrimp (preferably wild—check for when it's on sale) in the freezer for whenever the spirit moves you.

Ingredients
1 tablespoon extra-virgin olive oil
1–2 cloves garlic, minced
½ teaspoon red pepper flakes (optional)
1 pound shrimp, thawed, peeled, deveined, and dried
5 medium-sized zucchinis, spiralized
½ cup sliced red bell peppers and/or halved cherry tomatoes
½–1 cup pesto

Preparation
1. Heat the olive oil over medium heat. Add the garlic, and, if you like, red pepper flakes, and cook for 30 seconds. Add the shrimp. Cook the shrimp for 5 to 8 minutes, just until fully cooked and pink. Transfer the shrimp to a clean bowl or platter and set aside.
2. Add zucchini noodles to the same pan and sauté for 60 seconds over medium heat until just tender.
3. Plate the zucchini, shrimp, and bell pepper. Top with pesto. Alternatively, toss the shrimp, zucchini noodles, pepper slices, and pesto together in a bowl.

Note

Here's another way to prepare this dish: grill the shrimp on skewers over medium heat for 2 minutes on each side, or until just cooked. Microwave the zucchini noodles in a bowl with a tablespoon of water for 60 seconds. Drain. Plate or toss as above.

This is a good dish for piling on vegetables: steamed broccoli florets, broccolini, or asparagus, for example.

Sometimes, even though the spiralized zucchini *looks* like pasta, you still really do want *pasta*. Feel free to use two parts spiralized zucchini with one part cooked whole wheat pasta. It's still healthy.

SAUCES, DIPS & SALAD DRESSINGS

Chimichurri Sauce

Chimichurri is an uncooked sauce from Argentina that is traditionally served with grilled meats. We love this sauce on fish, which we've mentioned can sometimes be a little drab, and shellfish. It's also good with chicken and even on vegetables.

Ingredients

2–4 garlic cloves, peeled

⅓ cup coarsely chopped flat-leaf Italian parsley + 2 tablespoons, set aside

4 tablespoons balsamic or red wine vinegar

1–2 tablespoons oregano leaves (optional)

1–2 teaspoons crushed red pepper (optional)

½–¾ cup extra-virgin olive oil

Preparation

With the motor of a food processor running, drop in the garlic cloves and process until they're minced. Turn off the processor and add 1/3 cup parsley and vinegar, and, if you like, oregano and crushed pepper. Turn on the motor and process until smooth. With the motor running, add the olive oil in a gradual stream.

You can make this several hours ahead of time, or even refrigerate it overnight. Just before you serve it, chop up the reserved 2 tablespoons of parsley and add it to the sauce to brighten it up.

Miso Dressing

Miso is one of those superfoods that can be readily incorporated into all sorts of recipes. It has a wonderful umami taste; and since it is a fermented food, it's really great for your intestinal microbiome. This particular dressing is delicious on all sorts of things, including asparagus, broccoli, kale, and fish. It's also fantastic as a dip.

Ingredients
1 garlic clove, minced*
½ teaspoon grated or minced fresh ginger*
1–2 tablespoons white or yellow miso
2 tablespoons rice vinegar
2 tablespoons dark sesame oil
2 tablespoons canola oil
2 tablespoons plain yogurt
1 tablespoon fresh lime juice (optional)
Pinch cayenne (optional)

Preparation
Combine all the ingredients in a food processor. This dressing will keep for a week in your refrigerator.

Note
*If you put the garlic clove and ginger in the processor first, before any of the other ingredients, you can mince them that way to eliminate an extra preparation step.

Carrot Ginger Dressing

This is another easy, healthy, delicious, versatile recipe. It's adapted from a recipe from the incredibly knowledgeable food journalist and author Mark Bittman. The dressing is great on any kind of salad greens, as well as over grains. Kids love it.

Ingredients

2 carrots, cut into big chunks
1–2 tablespoons fresh ginger, peeled and cut into chunks
¼ cup rice vinegar
¼ cup white miso
2 tablespoons sesame oil
½ cup canola oil

Preparation

1. Finely chop the carrots and ginger in a food processor or blender (which will make a smoother texture).
2. Scrape down the sides, and add vinegar, miso, and sesame oil.
3. With the motor running, gradually add the canola oil. This will keep in the refrigerator for several days.

White Bean Dip

This recipe is so easy, healthy, and delicious. It is also wonderful as a spread on sandwiches.

Ingredients
2 (15-oz) cans white kidney or cannellini beans, rinsed and
    drained
2 tablespoons extra-virgin olive oil
1–2 garlic cloves, peeled
½ cup minced fresh basil or parsley or cilantro, or a combination
2 tablespoons fresh lemon juice
Salt and pepper to taste

Preparation
1. In a food processor, combine the beans, oil, and garlic. Process until smooth.
2. Add the basil, lemon juice, salt, and pepper. Process until blended.
3. Serve with crudités, such as jicama or bell pepper slices; carrot or celery sticks; or lightly steamed and cooled string beans, cauliflower, or broccoli.

AND OTHER DELIGHTS

Jae's Marinated Tofu

Serves 4

Janice—*Actually, I'm the one who chose this recipe. I'd always disliked the taste of tofu, but this recipe changed everything for me! You can bake it or sauté it. I kind of prefer the sautéed version because it's so easy to add in vegetables.*

Ingredients
1 (16-oz) package firm or extra firm tofu
1–2 cloves garlic, minced or grated
1 tablespoon peeled fresh gingerroot, minced or grated
1 tablespoon soy sauce or tamari
1 tablespoon fish sauce
3 tablespoons rice vinegar
2 tablespoons dry sherry or water
1 tablespoon maple syrup or honey

Preparation
1. Drain tofu and cut into 1-inch cubes.
2. Arrange the cubes in a single layer on several layers of paper towels. Cover with more layers of paper towels and top with something heavy (we like using a baking pan with a heavy skillet on top). Press the tofu for a least 20 minutes. You can put it in the refrigerator or leave it at room temperature.
3. Mix all the other ingredients together. Pour marinade over tofu and cover.
4. Refrigerate for 12 to 72 hours for maximum flavor.

To bake:

1. Place a sheet of parchment paper on a baking sheet. Arrange tofu in single layer on the sheet.
2. Save the marinade to use as a dipping sauce for later.
3. Bake at 350°F for 40 to 60 minutes, flipping tofu at least once during the process, until brown and slightly crispy.

To sauté:

1. Heat a skillet over high heat. Add enough oil for the pan, and wait 10 seconds or so for the oil to heat. Add the tofu and leave for a minute so it will brown. Then quickly stir-fry for another minute and transfer to a bowl. The tofu will crumble a bit as you do this.

Nora's Muffins

Makes 6 muffins

Here is a delicious muffin that's not just an excuse for eating cake in the morning. The ingredient list may look odd, but trust us—it's a wonderful and really filling treat. It's also great as an afternoon snack.

Janice—*I chose this recipe because Nora, my younger daughter, is the other light of my life and is also a wonderfully creative cook.*

Ingredients

½–1 cup old-fashioned oats

1 (15-oz) can chickpeas (garbanzo beans), rinsed and drained

½ cup unsweetened almond butter

¼ cup maple syrup

½ teaspoon salt

¼ teaspoon nutmeg

1 teaspoon vanilla (optional)*

¼ teaspoon cinnamon (optional)*

¼ teaspoon dried ginger (optional)*

¼ teaspoon baking soda (optional)**

Preparation

1. Preheat oven to 350°F. Fill muffin tin with paper liners.
2. Process the oats in the food processor a bit.
3. Add all the other ingredients to the food processor.
4. Pour batter into the lined muffin tins.
5. Bake for 25 to 30 minutes, until a toothpick comes out clean.

Note

*The vanilla, cinnamon, and ginger make the muffins a little sweeter. If you want a less sweet-tasting version, use nutmeg only.

**Omit baking soda if you want a somewhat denser texture.

Blueberry Yogurt Smoothie

Serves 2

Don't tell your kids that we included spinach in this—they won't notice the taste at all. (Even if the spinach makes it a little less pretty.) This recipe takes only a few minutes to make and is a great way to start the day.

Ingredients
1 cup fresh or frozen blueberries
Handful spinach
1 cup Greek yogurt
1 tablespoon honey or maple syrup
2 tablespoons old-fashioned oats

Preparation
Put all the ingredients in a blender and combine. Drink up!

Cathy's Quinoa Granola Snack

Janice—My friend Cathy is an extraordinary, inventive cook. I love these little gluten-free granola chunks. No, they're not salted caramel brownies, but they hit the spot if you want a snack that's sweet and that won't undermine your intentions to eat in a healthy, controlled way.

Ingredients

⅔ cup honey (heated until liquid)*
¼ cup coconut oil, melted, or any vegetable oil
½ teaspoon salt
¼ teaspoon cayenne pepper (optional)
2 cups toasted whole almonds, coarsely chopped
2 cups unsweetened coconut
1 cup rinsed quinoa, any color or mixed
1 cup old fashioned oatmeal
1 cup raw sunflower or pumpkin seeds
1 cup dried cherries or any other or mixture of dried fruit,
    chopped

Preparation

1. Preheat oven to 325°F.
2. Whisk together honey, oil, salt, and pepper in a large bowl.
3. Add the rest of the ingredients, and mix together until everything is well coated.
4. Place mixture in a parchment-lined baking pan. Press down until even and well compressed. The tighter you compact it, the chunkier the granola will be.
5. Bake until golden, 50 to 60 minutes.
6. Remove and leave in the pan until completely cool, at least an hour.

7. When completely cool, break into pieces. Store in airtight container.

Note

*The safest way to heat honey is to put the honey in a glass jar and set it in a pot with water up to the level of the honey. Bring the water to a boil, let it sit a bit, and carefully remove the jar. You can also microwave honey, but it can spatter and cleanup is a true pain.

FAVORITE SNACKS

In Chapter 22, we talked about how we can't live without snacks. Here are some of our favorites.

Jae's Favorite Snacks

I like high-protein snacks. They're satisfying and filling.
- *Tuna, on top of spinach, on top of a whole-grain cracker*
- *Fruit dip made of a blended nut butter, yogurt, honey, and cinnamon*
- *Hard-boiled eggs, chopped avocado, bell peppers, and onion*
- *Chickpeas, avocado, and feta cheese*
- *Whole-grain toast topped with cottage cheese, sliced avocado, and tomato*
- *Cucumbers thinly sliced lengthwise into strips (I use a vegetable peeler or a mandoline), topped with sliced turkey, pesto, red pepper slices, and spinach. Then I roll up the whole thing and secure with a toothpick—perfect for travel!*

My other favorite snacks:
- *Cauliflower cut into thin slices, roasted, and eaten as "chips"*
- *Carrots are the perfect mindless snack. They have a sweetness and a crunch that I often want when I'm having a snack.*

Janice's Favorite Snacks

I have to have snacks with me pretty much all the time. I think it's more of an anxiety thing than a hunger thing. That means I need to prepare ahead of time so I don't go down a rabbit hole of mindlessness and poor choices. Here are some of my go-to friends that I might take along with me:

- *Red pepper slices*
- *Jicama sticks*
- *Carrot sticks*
- *Apple slices*
- *Clementines*
- *Bosc pear slices (the other varieties get bruised and mushy)*
- *Almonds, in a limited quantity. Yes, they're really healthy, but they also have many calories. I eat plain roasted ones, which are not something I crave, as opposed to the ones covered in salt or sugar.*
- *Plain yogurt and berries (along with seeds or chopped nuts) in a plastic container. I keep a supply of plastic spoons in my car to avoid heartbreak and cursing.*

HEALTHY FOOD SWAPS

Here is a list of Jae's go-to food swaps—that is, healthier versions of some of the foods she loves.

Jae—When I'm craving pizza, I know it's really just the tomato sauce and cheese combo that I want. That's when I make mushroom cap pizzas. Making the swap will help me avoid eating impulsively or feeling deprived, and I'll feel proud of my success. Here are some others:

- *In addition to portabella mushroom caps, I use cooked, riced cauliflower as substitutes for pizza crust.*
- *I add fresh lime juice on my salad instead of dressing—it works!*
- *When I make lasagna, I replace the pasta with long mandoline-sliced zucchini strips.*
- *I use plain yogurt as a base for dips instead of sour cream.*
- *I add cottage cheese to pancakes for more protein. And I put fruit, not syrup (or maybe just a tiny bit), on top.*
- *Instead of bread, I wrap turkey burgers with collard greens or other leafy greens.*
- *I substitute mashed avocado or hummus for butter or mayonnaise on sandwiches.*

Janice—Jae's "portabella pizza" swap drives the point home that it's important to have healthy food available on hand in the kitchen so you can make delicious, healthy choices whenever you need it.

Acknowledgments

When we first embarked on our collaboration, we assumed that by sharing our stories and experiences, and by conveying the latest scientific knowledge, we would naturally be successful in writing and publishing this book.

Fortunately for us, our naiveté was matched by the incredible assistance and support of so many people, and we're grateful to be able to thank many of them in writing. Specifically, we want to thank Kim Lim, our editor at Skyhorse Publishing; Justin Loeber and the rest of the team at Mouth Digital PR; and Tim Lee, professional skateboarder and photographer, and now medical student, who got us started with web design. We particularly want to publicly thank our agent, Joan Parker, who believed in us from the beginning.

Janice's Acknowledgments

I would also like to thank the advice and assistance I received from my GNO Posse (Janice Hillman, MD, Lisa Rosen, MD, and Ann Steiner, MD), along with (in alphabetical order) Brenda Buchanan, Joyce Grossman, Susan Isaacs, Rebecca Pearl, MD, Cynthia Shar, Julie Stockler, Paul Tapino, MD, John Vasudevan, MD, and Mike Young.

My many years as the clinical director of Women's Health at the Student Health Service at the University of Pennsylvania were immensely rewarding, both professionally and personally. My colleagues, too many to name individually, were immensely support-ive of me in too many ways to count. I miss them every day.

Finally, this book, as is everything in my life, is for my daughters, Joanna and Nora.

In memory of my husband, David, who loved me always, even when I was "fluffy."

Jae's Acknowledgments

I would also like to express my gratitude to all those in my support system who enabled me to be successful in this process—whether it was literally running beside me, cooking meals with me, or wel-coming me into their homes—and to those who continue to share their love, encouragement, and friendship with me. Special mentions to those who shared their thoughts, time, and emotional support throughout the years of my transformation, writing this book, and all the wonderful things that have come afterward: Viktorya, Juan, Jacob, Ally, Persephone, Morgan, Zabby, Sarah, Syd, Emma and Neil, the La Casa fam, Emily, and so many more. Thank you to Janice for believing in me and our book, and to Dan for your love and support.

References

Chapter 2

1   Hall KD, Kahan S. Maintenance of Lost Weight and Long-Term Management of Obesity. Med Clin N Am 2018; 102:183–97.
2   Franz MJ et al. Weight-loss outcomes: a systematic review and meta-analysis of weight-loss clinical trials with a minimum 1-year follow-up. J Am Diet Assoc 2007; 107:1755–67.
3   Wing RR, Phelan S. Long-term weight loss maintenance. Am J Clin Nutr 2005; 82(1 Suppl):222S-5S.
4   Brach, Tara. *Radical Acceptance: Embracing Your Life with the Heart of a Buddha.* New York: Bantam, 2000.

Chapter 3

1   Butryn ML et al. Behavioral treatment of obesity. Psychiatr Clin N Am. 2011; 34(4):841–59.
2   Beck, Judith. *The Complete Beck Diet for Life: The Five-Stage Program for Permanent Weight Loss.* Birmingham: Oxmoor House, 2007.

Chapter 4

1   Pollan, Michael. *In Defense of Food: An Eater's Manifesto.* New York: Penguin Press, 2008.
2   Mozaffarian D et al. Changes in diet and lifestyle and long-term weight gain in women and men. N Engl J Med 2011; 364:2392–404.
3   Bertoia ML et al. Changes in intake of fruits and vegetables and weight change in United States men and women followed for up to 24 years: analysis from three prospective cohort studies. PLoS Med 2015; 12(9):e1001878.
4   Power ML, Schulkin J. *The Evolution of Obesity.* Baltimore: Johns Hopkins U Press, 2009.

5   Kearns CE et al. Sugar industry and coronary heart disease research: a historical analysis of internal industry documents. JAMA Int Med doi:10.1001/jamainternmed 2016:E1–E6.

6   Gross LS. Increased consumption of refined carbohydrates and the epidemic of type 2 diabetes in the United States; an ecologic assessment. Am J Clin Nutr 2004; 79(5):774–9.

7   Moss, Michael. *Salt, Sugar, Fat: How the Food Giants Hooked Us.* New York: Random House, 2013.

8   Gearhardt AN et al. Neural correlates of food addiction. Arch Gen Psychiatry 2011; 68(8):808–16.

9   Kessler, David. *The End of Overeating: Taking Control of the Insatiable American Appetite.* New York: Rodale, 2009.

10 Ludwig DS. Lifespan Weighed Down by Diet. JAMA 2016; 315(21):2269–70.

11 Hingle MD et al. Alignment of children's food advertising with proposed federal guidelines. Am J Prev Med 2015; 48(6):707–13.

12 Yilmaz Z et al. Supplements for diabetes mellitus: a review of the literature. J Pharm Pract 2017; 30(6):631–8.

13 Ebbeling CB et al. Effects of a low-glycemic load vs low fat diet in obese young adults: a randomized trial. JAMA 2007; 2092–102.

14 Wolever TMS et al. The glycemic index: methodology and clinical implications. Am J Clin Nutr 1991; 54:846–54.

15 Esposito K et al. A journey into a Mediterranean diet and type 2 diabetes: a systematic review with meta-analyses. BMJ Open 2015; 5(8):e008222.

16 Gross LS. Increased consumption of refined carbohydrates and the epidemic of type 2 diabetes in the United States; an ecologic assessment. Am J Clin Nutr 2004; 79(5):774–9.

17 Augustin LSA et al. Glycemic index, glycemic load and glycemic response: an international scientific consensus summit from the International Carbohydrate Quality Consortium (ICQC). Nutr, Metab & Cardiovasc Dis 2015; 25:795–815.

18 Mirrahimi A et al. Associations of glycemic index and load with coronary heart disease events: a systematic review and meta-analysis of prospective cohorts. J Am Heart Assoc 2012; 1:e000752.

19 Feinman RD et al. Dietary carbohydrate restriction as the first approach in diabetes management: critical review and evidence base. Nutrition 2015; 31(1):1–13.

20 Jacka FN et al. Western diet is associated with a smaller hippocampus: a longitudinal investigation. BMC Medicine 2015; 13:215.

21 Shapiro H et al. Personalized microbiome-based approaches to metabolic syndrome management and prevention. J Diab 2017; 9(3):226–36.

22 Tilg H, Adolph TE. Influence of the human intestinal microbiome in obesity and metabolic dysfunction. Curr Opin Pediatr 2015; 27(4):496–501.

23 Payne AN et al. Gut microbial adaptation to dietary consumption of fructose, artificial sweeteners and sugar alcohols: implications for host-microbe interactions contributing to obesity. Obes Rev 2012; 13:799–809.

24 D'Aversa F et al. Gut microbiota and metabolic syndrome. Intern Emerg Med 2013; 8 Suppl 1:S11–15.

25 Lynch SV, Pedersen O. The human intestinal microbiome in health and disease. N Engl J Med 2016; 375:2369–79.

26 Sherwin E. A gut (microbiome) feeling about the brain. Curr Opin Gastroent 2016; 32(2):96–102.

27 Collins S, Reid G. Distant site effects of ingested prebiotics. Nutrients 2016; 8(9): 523.

28 Martinez KB. Western diets, gut dysbiosis, and metabolic diseases: Are they linked? Gut Microbes 2017; 8(2):130–142.

29 De Filippis F et al. High-level adherence to a Mediterranean diet beneficially impacts the gut microbiota and associated metabolome. Gut 2016; 65(11):1812–8.

30 Anhe FF et al. Gut microbiota dysbiosis in obesity-linked metabolic diseases and prebiotic potential of polyphenol-rich extracts. Curr Obes Rep 2015; 4(4):389–400.

31 Distrutti E et al. Gut microbiota role in irritable bowel syndrome: New therapeutic strategies. World J Gastroent 2016; 22(7):2219–41.

32 Nishida A et al. Gut microbiota in the pathogenesis of inflammatory bowel disease. Clin J Gastroenterol 2018; 11(1):1–10.

33 Kaczmarek JL et al. Time of day and eating behaviors are associated with the composition and function of the human gastrointestinal microbiota. Am J Clin Nutr 2017; 106:1220–31.

34 Bo S et al. Consuming more of daily caloric intake at dinner predisposes to obesity: a 6-year population-based prospective cohort study. PLOS ONE 2014; 9:e108467.

35 Grund A et al. Increased risk of breast cancer associated with long-term shift work in Canada. Occup Environ Med 2013; 70:831–8.

36 Yamaguchi M et al. Relationship of dietary factors and habits with sleep-wake regularity. Asia Pac J Clin Nutr 2013; 22:457–65.

37 Reid KJ et al. Meal timing influences daily caloric intake in healthy adults. Nutr Res 2014; 930–5.

38 Heilbronn LK et al. Alternate-day fasting in nonobese subjects: effects on body weight, body composition, and energy metabolism. Am J Clin Nutr 2005; 81:69–73.

39 Varady KA. Impact of intermittent fasting on glucose homeostasis. Curr Opin Clin Nutr & Metab Care 2016; 19(4):300–2.

40 Appleion KM, Baker S. Distraction, not hunger is associated with lower perceived work performance on fast compared to non-fast days during intermittent fasting. J Hlth Psychol 2015; 20:702–11.

41 Headland M et al. Weight-loss outcomes: a systematic review and meta-analysis of intermittent energy restriction trials lasting a minimum of 6 months. Nutrients 2016; 8:354.

42 Blomquist C et al. Attenuated low-grade inflammation following long-term dietary intervention in postmenopausal women with obesity. Obesity 2017; 25(5):892–900.

43 David LA et al. Diet rapidly and reproducibly alters the human gut microbiome. Nature 2014; 505(7484):559–63.

44 Pannaraj PS et al. Association between breast milk bacterial communities and establishment and development of the infant gut microbiome. JAMA Pediatr 2017; doi:10.1001/jamapediatrics.2017.0378.

45 Tilg H, Adolph TE. Influence of the human intestinal microbiome in obesity and metabolic dysfunction. Curr Opin Pediatr 2015; 27(4):496–501.

46 Anhe FF et al. Gut microbiota dysbiosis in obesity-linked metabolic diseases and prebiotic potential of polyphenol-rich extracts. Curr Obes Rep 2015; 4(4):389–400.

47 Linares DM et al. Beneficial microbes: the pharmacy in the gut. Bioeng 2016; 7(1):11–20.

48 Martinez KB. Western diets, gut dysbiosis, and metabolic diseases: Are they linked? Gut Microbes 2017; 8(2):130–142.

49 Parker E et al. Probiotics and gastrointestinal conditions: An overview of evidence from the Cochrane Collaboration. Nutrition 2018; 45:125–134.e11.

50 Martinez KB. Western diets, gut dysbiosis, and metabolic diseases: Are they linked? Gut Microbes 2017; 8(2):130–142.

Chapter 5

1 Bertoia ML et al. Changes in Intake of Fruits and Vegetables and Weight Change in United States Men and Women Followed for Up to 24 Years: Analysis from Three Prospective Cohort Studies. PLoS Med 2015; 12(9):e1001878.

2 Bellavia et al. Fruit and vegetable consumption and all-cause mortality: a dose-response analysis. Am J Clin Nutr 2013; 98:454–9.

3 Limon-Miro AT et al. Dietary Guidelines for Breast Cancer Patients: A Critical Review. Adv Nutr 2017; 8(4):613–623.

4 Dacosta Christopher, Bao Y. The role of microRNAs in the chemopreventive activity of sulforaphane from cruciferous vegetables. Nutrients 2017; 9(8).

5 Abbaoui B et al. The impact of cruciferous vegetable isothiocyanates on histone acetylation and histone phosphorylation in bladder cancer. J Proteomics 2017; 156:94–103.

6 Hu J et al. Intake of cruciferous vegetables is associated with decreased ovarian cancer: a meta-analysis. Asia Pacif Clin Nutr 2015; 24(1):101–9.

7 Silva FM et al. Fiber intake and glycemic control in patients with type 2 diabetes mellitus: a systematic review with meta-analysis of randomized controlled trials. Nutr Rev 2013; 71(12):790–801.

8 Threapleton DE et al. Dietary fibre intake and risk of cardiovascular disease: systematic review and meta-analysis. BMJ 2013; (347): f6879.

9 Farvid MS et al. Dietary fiber intake in young adults and breast cancer risk. Pediatrics 2016; 137:1–11.

10 Weickert MO, Pfeiffer AFH. Impact of dietary fiber consumption on insulin resistance and the prevention of type 2 diabetes. J Nutr 2018; 148(1):7–12.

11 Ricker MA, Haas WC. Anti-inflammatory diet in clinical practice: a review. Nutr Clin Pract 2017; 32(3):318–25.

12 Ekmekcioglu C et al. Red meat, diseases, and healthy alternatives: A critical review. Crit Rev Food Sci Nutr 2018; 58(2):247–61.

13 Ebbeling CB et al. Effects of dietary composition on energy expenditure during weight-loss maintenance. JAMA 2012; 307(24):2627–34.

14 Siri-Tarino PW et al. Meta-analysis of prospective cohort studies evaluating the association of saturated fat with cardiovascular disease. Am J Clin Nutr 2010; 91:535–46.

15 Dehghan M et al. Associations of fats and carbohydrate intake with cardiovascular disease and mortality in 18 countries from five continents (PURE): a prospective cohort study. Lancet 2017; 390: 2050–62.

16 Mozaffarian D. Food and weight gain: time to end our fear of fat. Lancet Diabetes Endocrinol 2016; 4(8):633–5.

17 Wang DD et al. Association of specific dietary fats with total and cause-specific mortality. JAMA Intern Med 2016; 176(8):1134–45.

18 Golomb BA, Bui AK. A fat to forget: trans fat consumption and memory. PLoS ONE 2015; 10(6):e0128129.

19 Chowdhury R et al. Trans fatty acid isomers in mortality and incident coronary heart disease risk. J Am Heart Assoc 2014; 3(4).

20 Rautiainen S et al. Dairy consumption in association with weight change and risk of becoming overweight or obese in middle-aged and older women: a prospective cohort study. Am J Clin Nutr 2016; 103(4):979–88.

21 Mozaffarian D et al 2010. Effects on coronary heart disease of increasing polyunsaturated fat in place of saturated fat: a systematic review and meta-analysis of randomized controlled trials. PloS Medicine 2010; 7(3):1–10.

22 Cruz-Ten C et al. Dietary fat modifies the post-prandial inflammatory state in subjects with metabolic syndrome: the LIPGENE study. Mol Nutr Food Res 2012; 56:854–65.

23 Widmer RJ et al. The Mediterranean diet, its components, and cardiovascular disease. Am J Medicine 2015; 128:229–38.

24 Wu S et al. Omega-3 fatty acids intake and risks of dementia and Alzheimer's disease: a meta-analysis. Neurosci Biobehav Rev 2015; 48:1–9.

25 Gil A, Gil F. Fish, a Mediterranean source of n-3 PUFA: benefits do not justify limiting consumption. Br J Nutr 2014; 113:858–67.

26 Menon S 2016 www.nrdc.org/stories/mercury-guide.

27 Aung T et al. Associations of Omega-3 Fatty Acid Supplement Use With Cardiovascular Disease Risks. JAMA Cardiol 2018; 3(3):225–34.

28 Halton TL et al. Low-carbohydrate-diet score and the risk of coronary heart disease in women. N Engl J Med 2006; 355:1991–2002.

29 Larsson SC, Orsini N. Red meat and processed meat consumption and all-cause mortality: a meta-analysis. Am J Epidemiol 2013; 179(3):282–9.

30 Pan A et al. Red meat consumption and mortality. Arch Intern Med 2012; 172(7):555–63.

31 Knaus W. Perspectives on pasture versus indoor feeding of dairy cows. J Sci Food Agric 2016; 96(1):9–17.

32 Wu J et al. Dietary Protein Sources and Incidence of Breast Cancer: A Dose-Response Meta-Analysis of Prospective Studies. Nutrients 2016; 8(11).

33 Clayton ZS et al. Egg consumption and heart health: A review. Nutrition 2017 37:79–85.

34 Serra-Majem L, Bautista-Castano I. Relationship between bread and obesity. Br J Nutr 2015; 113:S29–35.

35 Mozaffarian D. Dietary and policy priorities for cardiovascular disease, diabetes, and obesity. Circulation 2016; 133:187–225.

36 Scharf RJ et al. Longitudinal evaluation of milk type consumed and weight status in preschoolers. Arch Dis Child 2013; 98:335–40.

37 Berkey CS et al. Milk, dairy fat, dietary calcium, and weight gain: a longitudinal study of adolescents. Arch Pediatr Adolesc Med 2005; 159:543–50.

38 Ludwig DS, Willett WC. Three daily servings of reduced-fat milk: an evidence-based recommendation? JAMA Pediatr 2013; 167(9):788–9.

39 Wong JMW et al. Effects of advice to drink 8 cups of water per day in adolescents with overweight or obesity: a randomized clinical trial. JAMA Pediatr 2017; 17(5):e170012.

40 Muckelbauer R et al. Association between water consumption and body weight outcomes: a systematic review. Am J Clin Nutr 2013; 98(2):282–99.

41 Artero A et al. The impact of moderate wine consumption on health. Maturitas 2015; 80(1):3–13.

42 Kunzmann AT et al. The association of lifetime alcohol use with mortality and cancer risk in older adults: A cohort study. PLoS Med 15(6): e1002585.

43 Katzke VA et al. Lifestyle and cancer risk. Cancer J 2015; 21(2):104–10.

44 Bagnardi V et al. Does drinking pattern modify the effect of alcohol on the risk of coronary heart disease? Evidence from a meta-analysis. J Epidemiol Community Health 2008; 62:615–9.

45 Mozaffarian D. Dietary and policy priorities for cardiovascular disease, diabetes, and obesity. Circulation 2016; 133:187–225.

46 Christensen L. Craving for sweet carbohydrate and fat-rich foods. Possible triggers and impact on nutritional intake. Nutr Bull 2007; 32:43–51.

47 Cogswell ME et al. Dietary sodium and cardiovascular disease risk—measurement matters. N Engl J Med 2016; 375:580–86.

48 Bolhuis DP et al. Salt Promotes Passive Overconsumption of Dietary Fat in Humans. J Nutr 2016; 146(4):838–5.

Chapter 6

1   Taubes, Gary. The Case Against Sugar. New York: Alfred A. Knopf, 2016.

2   Appelhans BM et al. Beverages contribute extra calories to meals and daily energy intake in overweight and obese women. Physiol & Behav 2013; 122:129–33.

3   Jastreboff A et al. Altered brain response to drinking glucose and fructose in obese adolescents. Diabetes 2016; 65(7):1929–39.

4   Huang M et al. Artificially sweetened beverages, sugar-sweetened beverages, plain water, and incident diabetes mellitus in postmenopausal women: the prospective Women's Health Initiative observational study. Am J Clin Nutr 2017; 106:614–22.

5   Wolf AM, Woodworth KA. Obesity prevention: recommended strategies and challenges. Am J Medicine 2009; 122:S19–S23.

6   Mozaffarian D et al. Changes in diet and lifestyle and long-term weight gain in women and men. N Engl J Med 2011; 364:2392–404.

7   Ludwig DS. Examining the health effects of fructose. JAMA 2013; 310(1):33–4.

8   Bray GA et al. Consumption of high-fructose corn syrup in beverages may play a role in the epidemic of obesity. Am J Clin Nutr 2004; 79:537–43.

9   Tucker KL et al. Colas, but not other carbonated beverages, are associated with low bone mineral density in older women: The Framingham Osteoporosis Study. Am J Clin Nutr 2006; 84(4):936.

10 Rosinger A et al. Sugar-sweetened beverage consumption among U.S. Adults, 2011–2014. NCHS Data Brief 2017; (270):1–8.

11 Payne AN et al. Gut microbial adaptation to dietary consumption of fructose, artificial sweeteners and sugar alcohols: implications for host-microbe interactions contributing to obesity. Obes Rev 2012; 13:799–809.

12 Schillinger D et al. Do sugar-sweetened beverages cause obesity and diabetes? Industry and the manufacture of scientific controversy. Ann Intern Med 2016; 165(12):895–7.

13 Aaron DG, Siegel MB. Sponsorship of National Health Organizations by Two Major Soda Companies. Am J Prev Med 2017; 52(1):20–30.

14 Boyland EJ et al. Advertising as a cue to consume: a systematic review and meta-analysis of the effects of acute exposure to unhealthy food and nonalcoholic beverage advertising on intake in children and adults. Am J Clin Nutr 2016; 102(3):519–33.

15 Powell LM, Maciejewsi ML. Taxes and sugar-sweetened beverages. JAMA 2018; 319(3):229–30.

16 Heyman MB, Abrams SA. Fruit juice in infants, children, and adolescents: current recommendations. Pediatrics 2017; 139(6)e20170967.

17 Stanhope KL et al. Consuming fructose-sweetened, not glucose-sweetened, beverages increases visceral adiposity and lipids and decreased insulin sensitivity in overweight/obese humans. J Clin Invest 2009; 119:1332–4.

18 Madjd A et al. Beneficial effects of replacing diet beverages with water on type 2 diabetic obese women following a hypo-energetic diet: A randomized, 24-week clinical trial. Diab Obes Metab 2017; 19(1):125–32.

19 Zhu Y et al. Maternal consumption of artificially sweetened beverages during pregnancy, and offspring growth through 7 years of age: a prospective cohort study. Intl J Epidemiol 2017; 1–10.

20 Mozaffarian D. Dietary and policy priorities for cardiovascular disease, diabetes, and obesity. Circulation 2016; 133:187–225.

21 Sylvetsky AC et al. Understanding the metabolic and health effects of low-calorie sweeteners: methodological considerations and implications for future research. Rev Endocr Metab Disord 2016; 17:187–94.

22 Suez J et al. Artificial sweeteners induce glucose intolerance by altering the gut microbiota. Nature 2014; 514(7521):181–6.

23 Pase MP et al. Sugar- and Artificially Sweetened Beverages and the Risks of Incident Stroke and Dementia. Stroke 2017; STROKEAHA.116.016027.

24 Hedrick V et al. Dietary quality changes in response to a sugar-sweetened beverage-reduction intervention: results from the Talking Health randomized controlled clinical trial. Am J Clin Nutr 2017; 105(4):824–33.

Chapter 8

1 Mozaffarian D. Dietary and policy priorities for cardiovascular disease, diabetes, and obesity. Circulation 2016; 133:187–225.

2 Grosso G et al. Beneficial effects of the Mediterranean diet on metabolic syndrome. Current Pharmaceutical Design 2014; 20(3):5039–44.

3 Artero A et al. The impact of moderate wine consumption on health. Maturitas 2015; 80(1):3–13.

4 Romaguera D et al. Adherence to the Mediterranean diet is associated with lower abdominal adiposity in European men and women. J Nutr 2009; 139(9):1728–37.

5 De Daniele N et al. Body composition changes and cardiometabolic benefits of a balanced Italian Mediterranean Diet in obese patients with metabolic syndrome. Acta Diabetol 2013; 50(3):409–16.

6 De Filippis F et al. High-level adherence to a Mediterranean diet beneficially impacts the gut microbiota and associated metabolome. Gut 2016; 65(11):1812–21.

7 Casas R et al. The immune protective effect of the Mediterranean diet against chronic low-grade inflammatory diseases. Endocr Metab Immune Disord Drug Targets 2014; 14(4):245–54.

8 Steckhan N et al. Effects of different dietary approaches on inflammatory markers in patients with metabolic syndrome: a systematic review and meta-analysis. Nutr 2016; 32:338–48.

9 Olivero F et al. How the Mediterranean diet and some of its components modulate inflammatory pathways in arthritis. Swiss Med Wkly 2015; 145:w14190.

10 Casazza, K et al. Myths, presumptions, and facts about obesity. N Engl J Med 2013; 368(23):2236–7.

11 Shai I et al. Weight loss with a low-carbohydrate, Mediterranean, or low-fat diet. N Engl J Med 2008; 359;229–41.

12 Estruch R et al. Primary prevention of cardiovascular disease with a Mediterranean diet supplemented with extra-virgin olive oil or nuts. N Engl J Med 2018; 378:e34.

13 Andersen CJ, Fernandez ML. Dietary strategies to reduce metabolic syndrome. Rev Endocr Metab Disord 2013; 14:241–54.

14 Esposito K et al. A journey into a Mediterranean diet and type 2 diabetes: a systematic review with meta-analysis. BMJ Open 2015; 5(8):e008222.

15 Martinez-Gonzalez MA et al. Benefits of the Mediterranean diet: insights from the PREDIMED study. Progress Cardiovasc Dis 2015; 58(1):50–60.

16 Widmer RJ et al. The Mediterranean diet, its components, and cardio-vascular disease. Am J Medicine 2015; 128:229–38.

17 Tektonidis TG et al. A Mediterranean diet and risk of myocardial infarction, heart failure and stroke: A population-based cohort study. Atherosclerosis 2015; 243(1):93–8.

18 Estruch R et al. Primary prevention of cardiovascular disease with a Mediterranean diet supplemented with extra-virgin olive oil or nuts. N Engl J Med 2018; 378:e34.

19 Lu,Y et al. Metabolic mediators of the effects of body-mass index, overweight, and obesity on coronary heart disease and stroke: a pooled analysis of 97 prospective cohorts with 1.8 million participants. Lancet 2014; 383:970–83.

20 Toledo E et al. Mediterranean diet and invasive breast cancer risk among women at high cardiovascular risk in the PREDIMED trial. JAMA intern Med 2015; 175(11):1752–60.

21 Barak Y, Fridman D. Impact of Mediterranean diet on cancer: focused literature review. Cancer Genomics Proteomics 2017; 14(6):403–8.

22 Garcia-Tora M et al. Obesity, metabolic syndrome and Mediterranean diet: impact on depression outcome. J Affective Disorders 2016; 194:105–8.

23 Anastasiou C et al. Mediterranean diet and cognitive health: Initial results from the Hellenic Longitudinal Investigation of Ageing and Diet. PLoS ONE 2017; 12(8):e0182048.

24 Feart C et al. Mediterranean diet and cognitive health: an update on available knowledge. Curr Opinion Clin Nutr & Metab Care 2015; 18(1):51–62.

25 Gu Y et al. Mediterranean diet and brain structure in a multiethnic elderly cohort. Neurol 2015; 85:1744–51.

26 Valls-Pedret C et al. Mediterranean diet and age-related cognitive decline: a randomized clinical trial. JAMA intern Med 2015; 175(7):1094–1103.

27 Serebrakian AT et al. Weight loss over 48 months is associated with reduced progression of cartilage T2 relaxation time values: data from the osteoarthritis initiative. J Magn Imaging 2015; 41(5):1272–80.

28 Dario AB et al. The relationship between obesity, low back pain, and lumbar disc degeneration when genetics and the environment are considered: a systematic review of twin studies. Spine 2015; 15(5):1106–17.

29 Koonce RC, Bravman JT. Obesity and osteoarthritis: More than just wear and tear. J Am Acad Orthop Surg 2013; 21(3):161–9.

30 Knoops KT et al. Mediterranean diet, lifestyle factor, and 10-year mortality in elderly European men and women: the HALE project. JAMA 2004; 292(2):1433–9.

31 Power ML, Schulkin J. *The Evolution of Obesity*. Baltimore: Johns Hopkins University Press, 2009.

Chapter 9

1 Jansen A et al. From lab to clinic: extinction of cued cravings to reduce overeating. Physiol & Behav 2016; 162:174–80.

2 Ferriday D, Brunstrom JM. "I just can't help myself": effects of food-cue exposure in overweight and lean individuals. Int J Obes 2011; 35(1):142–9.

3 Boswell RG, Kober H. Food cue reactivity and craving predict eating and weight gain: a meta-analytic review. Obes Rev 2016; 17:159–77.

Chapter 11

1 Butryn ML et al. Behavioral treatment of obesity. Psychiatr Clin N Am 2011; 34(4):841–59.

2 Troop NA et al. Expressive writing, self-criticism, and self-reassurance. Psychol Psychother 2013; 86(4):374–86.

3 Testa RJ, Brown RT. Self-regulatory theory and weight-loss maintenance. J Clin Psychol Med Settings 2015; 22:54–63.

4 Sato AF, Fahrenkamp AJ. From bench to bedside: understanding stress-obesity research within the context of translation to improve pediatric behavioral weight management. Ped Clin No Amer 2016; 63(3):401–23.

Chapter 12

1 Ahern AL et al. Participants' explanatory model of being overweight and their experiences of 2 weight loss interventions. Ann Fam Med 2013; 11(3):251–7.

Chapter 13

1 Benard M et al. Association between Impulsivity and Weight Status in a General Population. Nutrients 2017; 9(3).

2 Filbey F, Yezhuvath U. A multimodal study of impulsivity and body weight: Integrating behavioral, cognitive, and neuroimaging approaches. Obesity 2017; 25(1):147–54.

3 Butryn ML et al. Behavioral treatment of obesity. Psychiatr Clin N Am. 2011; 34(4):841–59.

Chapter 14

1 Dallman MF. Stress-induced obesity and the emotional nervous system. Trends Endocrinol Metab 2010; 21:159–65.

2 Adam TC, Epel ES. Stress, eating and the reward system. Physiol Behav 2007; 91:449–58.

3 Lennerz BS, et al. Effects of dietary glycemic index on brain regions related to reward and craving in men. Am J Clin Nutr 2013; 98:641–7.

4 Geiker NRW et al. Does stress influence sleep patterns, food intake, weight gain, abdominal obesity and weight loss interventions and vice versa? Obes Rev 2018; 19(1):81–97.

5 Born J et al. Acute stress and food-related reward activation in the brain during food choice during eating in the absence of hunger. Int J Obes (Lond) 2010; 34:172–81.

6 Sinha R, Jastreboff AM. Stress as a common risk factor for obesity and addiction. Biol Psychiatry 2013; 73:827–35.

7 Aschbacher K et al. Chronic stress increases vulnerability to diet-related abdominal fat, oxidative stress, and metabolic risk. Psychoneuroendocrin 2014; 46:14–22.

8 Grandner M et al. Sleep duration and diabetes risk: population trends and potential mechanisms. Curr Diab Rep 2016; 16(11):106.

9 Warne JP. Shaping the stress response: interplay of palatable food choices, glucocorticoids, insulin and abdominal obesity. Mol Cell Endocrinol 2009; 300(1–2):137–46.

10 Tryon MS et al. Chronic stress exposure may affect the brain's response to high-calorie food cues and predispose to obesogenic eating habits. Physiol Behav 2013; 120:233–42.

11 Himmelstein MS et al. The weight of stigma: cortisol reactivity to manipulated weight stigma. Obesity 2015; 23:368–74.

12 Vanaelst B et al. The association between childhood stress and body composition, and the role of stress-related lifestyle factors—cross-sectional findings from the baseline ChiBS survey. Int J Behav Med 2014; 21:292–301.

13 Harris JL et al. US Food Company Branded Advergames on the Internet: children's exposure and effects on snack consumption. J Child Media 2012; 651–68.

14 Wonderlich-Tierney AL et al. Food-related advertisements and food intake among adult men and women. Appetite 2013; 71:57–62.

15 Gearhardt AN et al. Relation of obesity to neural activation in response to food commercials. Social Cognitive & Affective Neurosci 2014; 9(7):932–8.

16 Boswell RG, Kober H. Food cue reactivity and craving predict eating and weight gain: a meta-analytic review. Obes Rev 2016; 17:159–77.

17 Jansen A et al. Overweight children overeat after exposure to food cues. Eat Behav 2003; 4:197–209.

18 Jansen A et al. From lab to clinic: extinction of cued cravings to reduce overeating. Physiol & Behav 2016; 162:174–80.

19 Chao A et al. Stress, cortisol, and other appetite-related hormones: prospective prediction of 6-month changes in food cravings and weight. Obesity 2017; 25:713–20.

20 Yokum S, Stice E. Cognitive regulation of food craving; effects of three cognitive reappraisal strategies on neural response to palatable foods. Intl J Obes 2013; 37;1565–70.

21 Schulte EM et al. Which foods may be addictive? The roles of processing, fat content, and glycemic load. PLoS ONE 2015; 10(2):e0117959.

Chapter 15

1 Westbrook JI. Interruptions and multi-tasking: moving the research agenda in new directions. BMJ Qual Saf 2014; 23(11):877–9.

2 Mason AE et al. Reduced reward-driven eating accounts for the impact of a mindfulness-based diet and exercise intervention on weight loss:

Data from the SHINE randomized controlled trial. J. Appet 2016; 100:86–93.

3 Olson KL, Emery CF. Mindfulness and weight loss: a systematic review. Psychos Med 2015; 77 (1):59–67.

4 Paulson S et al. Becoming conscious: the science of mindfulness. Ann N Y Acad Sci 2013; 1303:87–104.

5 Crosswell AD et al. Effects of mindfulness training on emotional and physiologic recovery from induced negative affect. Psychoneuroendocrin 2017; 86:78–86.

6 Katterman SN et al. Mindfulness meditation as an intervention for binge eating, emotional eating, and weight loss: a systematic review. Eat Behav 2014; 15:197–204.

7 Boccia M et al. The meditative mind: a comprehensive meta-analysis of MRI studies. Biomed Res Int 2015:419808.

8 Winnebeck, E et al. Brief training in mindfulness meditation reduces symptoms in patients with a chronic or recurrent lifetime history of depression: A randomized controlled study. Behav Res Ther 2017; 99:124–30.

9 Holze BK et al. Mindfulness practice leads to increases in regional brain gray matter density. Psych Res 2011; 191(1):36–43.

Chapter 16

1 Schoenborn CA, Adams, PE. Health behaviors of adults: United States, 2005–2007. Vital and Health Stat Series 10, Data from the Natl Health Survey 2010:1–132.

2 Spaeth AM et al. Effects of experimental sleep restriction on weight gain, caloric intake and meal timing in healthy adults. Sleep 2013; 36:981–90.

3 Broussard JL et al. Elevated ghrelin predicts food intake during experimental sleep restriction. Obesity 2016; 24:132–138.

4 St.-Onge MP et al. Sleep restriction increases the neuronal response to unhealthy food in normal-weight individuals. Int J Obes 2014; 38:411–6.

5 Grandner MA et al. Sleep duration and diabetes risk: population trends and potential mechanisms. Curr Diab Rep 2016; 16(11):106.

6 Dulloo AG et al. Nutrition, movement and sleep behaviors: their interactions in pathways to obesity and cardiometabolic diseases. Obes Rev 2017; 18(suppl.1):3–6.

7   Ng W et al. Does intentional weight loss improve daytime sleepiness? A systematic review and meta-analysis. Obes Rev 2017; 18(4):460–75.

8   Naufel MF et al. Association Between Obesity and Sleep Disorders in Postmenopausal Women. Menopause 2018; 25(2):139–44.

9   Fatima Y et al. Sleep quality and obesity in young subjects: a meta-analysis. Obes Rev 2016; 17:1154–65.

10 Geiker NRW et al. Does stress influence sleep patterns, food intake, weight gain, abdominal obesity and weight loss interventions and vice versa? Obes Rev 2018; 19(1):81–97.

11 Ma N et al. How acute total sleep loss affects the attending brain: a meta-analysis of neuroimaging studies. Sleep 2015; 38(2):233.

12 Itani O et al. Short sleep duration and health outcomes: a systematic review, meta-analysis, and meta-regression. Sleep Med 2017; 32:246–56.

13 Owens JA, Weiss MR. Insufficient sleep in adolescents: causes and consequences. Minerva Pediatr 2017; 69(4):326–36.

14 https://www.cdc.gov/features/dsdrowsydriving/index.html.

15 Chapman CD et al. Acute sleep deprivation increases food purchasing in men. Obesity 2013; 21:E555–60.

16 Goel N et al. Circadian rhythms, sleep deprivation, and human performance. Prog Mol Biol Transl Sci 2013; 119:155.

17 Shimizu I et al. A role for circadian clock in metabolic disease. Hypertens Res 2016; 39(7):483–91.

18 McHill AW, Wright Jr KP. Role of sleep and circadian disruption on energy expenditure and in metabolic predisposition to human obesity and metabolic disease. Obes Rev 2017; 18(suppl 1):15–24.

19 Albrecht U. The circadian clock, metabolism and obesity. Obes Rev 2017; 18(suppl 1):25–33.

20 Horne J. The end of sleep: "sleep debt" versus biological adaptation of human sleep to waking needs. Biol Psychol 2011; 87(1):1. Epub 2010.

21 Mantua J, Spencer RMC. Exploring the nap paradox: are mid-day sleep bouts a friend or foe? Sleep Med 2017; 37:88–97.

22 Tasali E et al. The effects of extended bedtimes on sleep duration and food desire in overweight young adults: a home-based intervention. Appetite 2014; 80:220–4.

23 Alfaris N et al. Effects of a two-year behavioral weight loss intervention on obese individuals treated in a primary care practice. Obesity 2015; 23(3): 558–564.

REFERENCES

Chapter 17

1   Lee JS et al. Combined eating behaviors and overweight: Eating quickly, late evening meals, and skipping breakfast. Eat Behav 2016; 21:84–8.
2   Olson KL, Emery CF. Mindfulness and weight loss: a systematic review. Psychos Med 2015; 77(1):59–67.
3   Yokum S, Stice E. Cognitive regulation of food craving; effects of three cognitive reappraisal strategies on neural response to palatable foods. Intl J Obes 2013; 37:1565–70.
4   Schonberg T et al. Influencing food choices by training: evidence for modulation of frontoparietal control signals. J Cogn Neurosci 2014; 26(2):247–68.
5   Hare TA et al. Focusing attention on the health aspects of foods changes value signals in vmPFC and improves dietary choice. J Neurosci 2011; 31(30):11077–87.

Chapter 18

1   Kyu HH et al. Physical activity and the risk of breast cancer, colon cancer, diabetes, ischemic heart disease, and ischemic stroke events: systematic review and dose-response meta-analysis for the Global Burden of Disease Study 2013. BMJ 2016; 354:i3857.
2   Lear SA et al. The effect of physical activity on mortality and cardiovascular disease in 130,000 people from 17 high-income, middle-income, and low-income countries: the PURE study. Lancet 2017; 390:2643–54.
3   Rahman I et al. Relationship between physical activity and heart failure risk in women. Circ Heart Fail 2014; 7:877–81.
4   Moore SC et al. Association of leisure-time physical activity with risk of 26 types of cancer in 1.44 million adults. JAMA Intern med 2016; E1-E10.
5   Shaw E et al. Effects of physical activity on colorectal cancer risk among family history and body mass index subgroups: a systematic review and meta-analysis. BMC Cancer 2018; n18(1):71.
6   Friedenreich CM et al. Epidemiology and biology of physical activity and cancer recurrence. J Mol Med 2017; 95(10):1029–41.
7   Neil-Sztramko SE et al. Does obesity modify the relationship between physical activity and breast cancer risk? Breast Cancer Res Treat 2017; 166(2):367–81.

8   Clarke SF et al. Exercise and associated dietary extremes impact on gut microbial diversity. Gut 2014; 63:1913–20.

9   Abbasi J. Can exercise prevent knee osteoarthritis? JAMA 2017; 318(22):2169–71.

10 Zhao R et al. The effectiveness of combined exercise intervention for preventing postmenopausal bone loss: a systematic review and meta-analysis. J Orthopaed & Sports Phys Ther 2017; 47(4):241–51.

11 Peterson ND, Gordon PM. Resistance exercise for the aging adult: clinical implications and prescription guidelines. Am J Med 2011; 124(3):194–8.

12 Sherrington C et al. Exercise to prevent falls in older adults: an updated systematic review and meta-analysis. BJSM online 2017; 51(24):1750–8.

13 Lee T et al. Aerobic exercise interacts with neurotrophic factors to predict cognitive functioning in adolescents. Psychoneuroendocrin 2014; 39:214–24.

14 Prakash RS et al. Physical activity and cognitive vitality. Ann Rev Psychol 2015; 66:769–97.

15 Azizan A, Jusine M. Effects of behavioral and exercise program on depression and quality of life in community-dwelling older adults: a controlled, quasi-experimental study. J Gerontol Nurs 2016; 42(2):45–54.

16 Carter T et al. Exercise for adolescents with depression; valued aspects and perceived change. J Psychiatric Metal Hlth Nurs 2016; 23(1):37–44.

17 Azizan A, Jusine M. Effects of behavioral and exercise program on depression and quality of life in community-dwelling older adults: a controlled, quasi-experimental study. J Gerontol Nurs 2016; 42(2):45–54.

18 Carraca EV et al. The association between physical activity and eating self-regulation in overweight and obese women. Obes Facts 2013; 6:493–506.

19 Melanson EL. The effect of exercise on non-exercise physical activity and sedentary behavior in adults. Obes Rev 2017; 18(suppl 1):50–55.

20 Kwon S et al. Active lifestyle in childhood and adolescence prevents obesity development in young adulthood. Obes 2015; 23(12):2462–9.

21 Hankinson AL et al. Maintaining a high physical activity level over 20 years and weight gain. JAMA 2010; 304:2603.

22 Pronk NP. Combined Diet and Physical Activity Promotion Programs for Prevention of Diabetes: Community Preventive Services Task Force Recommendation Statement. Annals Int Med 2015; 163(6):465–8.

23 Manini TM et al. Daily activity energy expenditure and mortality among older adults. JAMA 2006; 296(20);171–9.

24 Villareal DT et al. Aerobic or Resistance Exercise, or Both, in Dieting Obese Older Adults. N Engl J Med 2017; 376:1943–55.

25 Kennedy AB et al. Fitness or fatness. Which is more important? JAMA 2018; 319(3):231–2.

26 US Department of Health and Human Services. 2008 Physical Activity Guidelines for Americans. https://health.gov/paguidelines/2008/pdf/paguide.pdf.

27 Turner TL, Stevinson C. Affective outcomes during and after high-intensity intensity exercise in outdoor green and indoor gym settings. Int J Environ Health Res 2017; 27(2):106–16.

28 Puett, R et al. Physical activity: does environment make a difference for tension, stress, emotional outlook, and perceptions of health status? J Phys Act Health 2014; 11(8):1503–11.

29 Lacharite-Lemieux M et al. Adherence to exercise and affective responses: comparison between outdoor and indoor training. Menopause 2015; 22(7):731–40.

30 Farrokhi S et al. The influence of continuous versus interval walking exercise on knee loading and pain in patients with knee osteoarthritis. Gait & Posture 2017; 56:129–33.

31 Goodpaster BH et al. The loss of skeletal muscle strength, mass, and quality in older adults: the health, aging and body composition study. J Gerontol Biol Sci Med Sci 2006; 61(10):1059–64.

32 Northey JM et al. Exercise interventions for cognitive function in adults older than 50: a systematic review with meta-analysis. Br J Sports Med 2018; 2017; 52(3):154–60.

33 Beavers KM et al. Effect of Exercise Type During Intentional Weight Loss on Body Composition in Older Adults with Obesity. Obesity 2017; (11):1823–1829.

34 Kutzner I et al. Does aquatic exercise reduce hip and knee joint loading? In vivo load measurements with instrumented implants. PLoSOne 2017; 12(3):e0171972.

35 Dong R et al. Is aquatic exercise more effective than land-based exercise for knee osteoarthritis. Medicine 2018 Dec; 97(52):e13823.

36 Cadmus-Bertram LA et al. Randomized Trial of a Fitbit-Based Physical Activity Intervention for Women. Am J Prev Med 2015; 49(3):414–8.

Chapter 22

1   Casazza, K et al. Myths, presumptions, and facts about obesity. N Engl J Med 2013; 368(23):2236–7.

2   Sievert K et al. Effect of breakfast on weight and energy intake: systematic review and meta-analysis of randomised controlled trials. BMJ 2019; 364:l42.

3   Sofer S et al. Greater Weight Loss and Hormonal Changes After 6 Months Diet With Carbohydrates Eaten Mostly at Dinner. Obesity 2011; 19(10):2006–14.

4   Jakubowicz D et al. High caloric intake at breakfast vs. dinner differentially influences weight loss of overweight and obese women. Obesity 2013; 21(12)2504–12.

5   Nas A et al. Impact of breakfast skipping compared with dinner skipping on regulation of energy balance and metabolic risk. Am J Clin Nutr 2017; 105(6):1351–61.

6   Karatzi K et al. Late-night-overeating is associated with smaller breakfast, breakfast skipping, and obesity in children: the Healthy Growth Study. Nutr 2017; 33:141–4.

7   Kranz S et al. High-protein and high-dietary fiber breakfasts result in equal feelings of fullness and better diet quality in low-income preschoolers compared with their usual breakfast. J Nutr 2017; 147(3):445–52.

Chapter 23

1   Butryn ML et al. Behavioral treatment of obesity. Psychiatr Clin N Am. 2011; 34(4):841–59.

2   Hollands CJ et al. Portion, package or tableware size for changing selection and consumption of food, alcohol and tobacco. Cochrane Database Syst Rev 2015; (9):CD011045. doi: 10.1002/1465.

Chapter 24

1   Anderson JW et al. Long-term weight-loss maintenance: a meta-analysis of US studies. Am J Clin Nutr 2001; 74(5):579–84.

2   Wing RR, Phelan S. Long-term weight loss maintenance. Am J Clin Nutr 2005; 82(1 Suppl):222S–5S.

3   Anastasiou CA et al. Weight regaining: From statistics and behaviors to physiology and metabolism. Metab 2105; 64(11):1395–1407.

4　Schwartz A, Doucet E. Relative changes in resting energy expenditure during weight loss: a systematic review. Obes Rev 2010; 11:531–47.

5　Sumithran P et al. Long-term persistence of hormonal adaptations to weight loss. N Engl J Med 2011; 365(17):1597–1604.

6　Polidori D et al. How strongly does appetite counter weight loss? Quantification of the feedback control of human energy intake. Obesity 2016; 24(11):2289–95.

7　Bray GA, Wadden TA. Improving long-term weight loss maintenance: can we do it? Obesity 2015; 23(1):2–3.

8　Hall KD, Kahan S. Maintenance of Lost Weight and Long-Term Management of Obesity. Med Clin N Am 2018; 102:183–97.

9　Martinez Steele E et al. Ultra-processed foods and added sugars in the US diet: evidence from a nationally representative cross-sectional study. BMJ open 2016; 6(3):e009892.

10　Puhl RM, Heuer CA. The Stigma of Obesity: A Review and Update. Obesity 2009; 17(5):941–64.

11　Volpp KG et al. Financial incentive-based approaches for weight loss: a randomized trial. JAMA 2008; 300(22):2631–37.

12　Melby CL et al. Attenuating the biologic drive for weight regain following weight loss: must what goes down always go back up? Nutrients 2017; 2(5):https://doi.org/10.3390/nu9050468.

13　Larsen TM et al. Diets with high or low protein content and glycemic index for weight-loss maintenance. N Engl J Med 2010; 363:2102–13.

14　Paddon-Jones D et al. Protein, weight management, and satiety. Am J Clin Nutr 2008; 87:1558S–61S.20.

15　van Baak M et al. Dietary intake of protein from different sources and weight regain, changes in body composition and cardiometabolic risk factors after weight loss: the DIOGenes Study. Nutrients 2017; 9(12).

16　John Hopkins Medicine. Protein Content of Common Foods. https://www.hopkinsmedicine.org/johns_hopkins_bayview/_docs/medical_services/bariatrics/nutrition_protein_content_common_foods.pdf.

17　Jakubowicz D, Barnea M, Wainstein J, Froy O. High caloric intake at breakfast vs. dinner differentially influences weight loss of overweight and obese women. Obesity 2013; 21:2504–12.

18　Jakubowicz D, Froy O, Wainstein J, Boaz M. Meal timing and composition influence ghrelin levels, appetite scores and weight loss maintenance in overweight and obese adults. Steroids 2012; 77:323–31.

19 Franz MJ et al. Weight-loss outcomes: a systematic review and meta-analysis of weight-loss clinical trials with a minimum 1-year follow-up. J Am Diet Assoc 2007;107:1755–67.

20 Greenway FL. Physiological adaptations to weight loss and factors favouring weight regain. Int J Obes 2015; 39(8:)1188–96.

21 Ochner CN et al. Treating obesity seriously: when recommendations for lifestyle change confront biological adaptations. Lancet Diab Endocrinol 2015; 3(4):232–34.

22 Soini S et al. Lifestyle-related factors associated with successful weight loss. Ann Med 2015; 47:88–93.

23 Pronk NP. Combined Diet and Physical Activity Promotion Programs for Prevention of Diabetes: Community Preventive Services Task Force Recommendation Statement. Ann Int Med 2015; 163(6):465–8.

24 Peterson ND et al. Dietary self-monitoring and long-term success with weight management. Obesity 2014; 22(9):1962–7.

25 Butryn ML et al. Behavioral treatment of obesity. Psychiatr Clin N Am. 2011; 34(4):841–59.

26 Ohsiek S, Williams M. Psychological factors influencing weight loss maintenance: an integrative literature review. J Amer Acad Nurse Pract 2011; 23:596–601.

27 Kozica S et al. Initiating and continuing behaviour change within a weight gain prevention trial: a qualitative investigation. Plos One/DOI 2015; 1–14.

28 Testa RJ, Brown RT. Self-regulatory theory and weight-loss maintenance. J Clin Psychol Med Settings 2015; 22:54–63.

29 Troop NA. The effect of current and anticipated body pride and shame on dietary restraint and caloric intake. Appetite 2016; 96:375–82.

Chapter 25

1 Lindeman, M et al. The effects of messages about the causes of obesity on disciplinary action decisions for overweight employees. J Psychol 2017; 151(4):345–58.

2 Phelan SM et al. Impact of weight bias and stigma on quality of care and outcomes for patients with obesity. Obes Rev 2015; 16:319–26.

3 Puhl RM, Heuer CA. The Stigma of Obesity: A Review and Update. Obesity 2009; 17(5):941–64.

4   Cheng HL et al. The Health Consequences of Obesity in Young Adulthood. Curr Obes Rep 2016; 5(1):30–7.

5   Puhl RM, Latner JD. Stigma, obesity, and the health of the nation's children. Psychol Bull 2007; 133:557-80.

6   Gearhardt AN et al. Obesity and public policy. Ann Rev Clin Psychol 2012; 8:405–30.

7   Puhl, RM et al. Experiences of weight teasing in adolescence and weight-related outcomes in adulthood: A 15-year longitudinal study. Prev Med 2017; 100:173–79.

8   Himmelstein MS et al. The weight of stigma: cortisol reactivity to manipulated weight stigma. Obesity 2015; 23:368–74.

9   Friedman KE et al. Weight stigmatization and ideological beliefs: relation to psychological functioning in obese adults. Obes Res 2005; 13:907-16.

10 Wang SS et al. The influence of the stigma of obesity on overweight individuals. Int J Obes Relat Metab Disord 2004; 28:1333-7.

11 Foster GD et al. Primary care physicians' attitudes about obesity and its treatment. Obes Res 2003; 11:1168–77,

12 Puhl RM et al. Obesity bias in training attitudes, beliefs, and observations among advanced trainees in professional health disciplines. Obesity 2014; 22(4):1008–15.

13 Phelan SM et al. Impact of weight bias and stigma on quality of care and outcomes for patients with obesity. Obes Rev 2015; 16:319–26.

14 Gay, Roxane. *Hunger: A Memoir of (My) Body.* New York: Harper Collins, 2017.

15 Gu W et al. Obesity-associated endometrial and cervical cancers. Front Biosci 2013; 5:1.

16 Pearl RL, Puhl RM. The distinct effects of internalizing weight bias: An experimental study. Body Image 2016; 17:38–42.

17 Puhl RM, Brownell K. Confronting and coping with weight stigma: an investigation of overweight and obese adults. Obesity 2006; 14:1802–15.

18 Dulloo AG, Montani JP. Pathways from dieting to weight regain, to obesity and to the metabolic syndrome: an overview. Obes Rev 2015; 16(Suppl. 1):1–6).

19 Vartanian LR, Novak SA. Internalized societal attitudes moderate the impact of weight stigma on avoidance of exercise. Obesity 2011; 19:757-62.

20 Pearl R et al. Differential effects of weight bias experiences and internalization on exercise among women with overweight and obesity. J Health Psychol 2012:1626–32.

21 Pearl R et al. Differential effects of weight bias experiences and internalization on exercise among women with overweight and obesity. J Health Psychol 2012:1626–32.

22 West, Lindy. *Shrill: Notes from a Loud Woman.* New York: Hachette, 2016.

Chapter 26

1 Flegal KM et al. Trends in obesity among adults in the United States, 2005 to 2014. JAMA 2016; 315(21):2284–91.

2 Mozaffarian D et al. Changes in diet and lifestyle and long-term weight gain in women and men. N Engl J Med 2011; 365:2392–2404.

3 Zheng Y et al. Associations of weight gain from early to middle adulthood with major health outcomes later in life. JAMA 2017; 318(3):255–69.

4 Aune D et al. Body mass index, abdominal fatness, and heart failure incidence and mortality: a systematic review and dose-response meta-analysis of prospective studies. Circulation 2016; 133(7):639–49.

5 Lu Y et al. Metabolic mediators of the effects of body-mass index, overweight, and obesity on coronary heart disease and stroke: a pooled analysis of 97 prospective cohorts with 1.8 million participants. Lancet 2014; 383:970–83.

6 Baldauff NH, Witchel SF. Polycystic ovarian syndrome in adolescent girls. Curr Opin Endocrin, Diab & Obes 2017; 24(1):56–66.

7 Morgante G et al. Therapeutic approach for metabolic disorders and infertility in women with PCOS. Gynecol Endocrinol 2018; 34(1):4–9.

8 Declerq E et al. Prepregnancy body mass index and infant mortality in 38 U.S. States, 2012–2013. Ob & Gyn 2016; 127(2):279–87.

9 Houghton LC et al. Maternal weight gain in excess of pregnancy guidelines is related to daughters being overweight 40 years later. Am J Obstet Gynecol 2016; 215:246–7.

10 Aune D et al. Maternal body mass index and the risk of fetal death, stillbirth, and infant death: a systematic review and meta-analysis. JAMA 2014; 311(15):1536–46.

11 Veronese, N et al. Combined associations of body weight and lifestyle factors with all cause and cause specific mortality in men and women: prospective cohort study. BMJ 2016; 355:i5855.

12 Kramer CK et al. Are metabolically healthy overweight and obesity benign conditions? A systematic review and meta-analysis. Ann Intern Med 2013; 159:758–69.

13 King DE et al. Turning back the clock: adopting a healthy lifestyle in middle age. Am J Med 2007; 120:598–603.

14 Blomquist C et al. Attenuated low-grade inflammation following long-term dietary intervention in postmenopausal women with obesity. Obesity 2017; 25(5):892–900.

15 Villreal DT et al. Weight loss, exercise, or both and physical function in obese older adults. N Eng J Med 2011; 364:1218–29.

16 Horie NC et al. Cognitive effects of intentional weight loss in elderly obese individuals with mild cognitive impairment. J Clin Endocrin Metab 2016; 10(3):1104–12.

17 Centers for Disease Control and Prevention. The Childhood Obesity Epidemic: Threats and Opportunities. https://www.cdc.gov/grand-rounds/pp/2010/20100617-childhood-obesity.html.

18 Cheng HL et al. The Health Consequences of Obesity in Young Adulthood. Curr Obes Rep 2016; 5(1):30–7.

19 Kit BK et al. Prevalence of and trends in dyslipidemia and blood pressure among US children and adolescents, 1999–2012. JAMA Pediatr 2015; 169(3):272–9.

20 Twig G et al. Body-mass index in 2.3 million adolescents and cardiovascular death in adulthood. N Engl J Med 2016; 374(25):2430–40.

21 Harris HR et al. An adolescent and early adulthood dietary pattern associated with inflammation and the incidence of breast cancer. Cancer Res 2017; 77(5):1179–87.

22 Smith SM et al. Musculoskeletal pain in overweight and obese children. Int J Obes 2014; 38(1):11–15.

23 Hutchins J et al. Type 2 diabetes in a 5-year-old and single center experience of type 2 diabetes in youth under 10. Pediatr Diab 2017; 18(7):674–7.

24 Puhl RM, Latner JD. Stigma, obesity, and the health of the nation's children. Psychol Bulletin 2007; 133(4):557–80.

25 Pronk NP. Combined Diet and Physical Activity Promotion Programs for Prevention of Diabetes: Community Preventive Services Task Force Recommendation Statement. Annals Int Med 2015; 163(6):465–8.

26 Altman M, Wilfley DE. Evidence update on the treatment of overweight and obesity in children and adolescents. J Clin Child & Adolesc Psych 2015; 44(4):521–37.

27 Harris HR et al. An adolescent and early adulthood dietary pattern associated with inflammation and the incidence of breast cancer. Cancer Res 2017; 77(5):1179–87.

28 Gravelle BL, Broyles M. Interventions of weight reduction and prevention in children and adolescents: update. Amer J Therapeutics 2015; 22(2):159–66.

29 Hollands CJ et al. Portion, package or tableware size for changing selection and consumption of food, alcohol and tobacco. Cochrane Database Syst Rev 2015; (9):CD011045. doi: 10.1002/1465.

30 Watts AW et al. Characteristics of a favorable weight status change from adolescence to young adulthood. J Adolesc Hlth 2016; 58(4):403–9.

Conclusion

1   Whitely, Kara Richardson. *Gorge: My Journey Up Kilimanjaro at 300 Pounds.* Berkeley, CA: Seal Press, 2015.

2   Ramsey, Drew. *Eat Complete: The 21 Nutrients That Fuel Brainpower, Boost Weight Loss, and Transform Your Health.* New York: Harper Collins, 2016.

Index

INDEX